COLORS of YOU

Lesson Plans for Teachers and Parents about Sex Education and Identity

Kristen Lilla, LCSW, CST, CSE, CSTS, CSES, and Christian Hoeger MA, MEd, LMHP

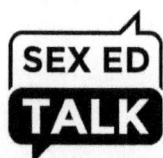

SEX ED
TALK

Sex Ed Talk LLC
Omaha, NE

Copyright 2023 by Kristen Lilla and Christian Hoeger. All rights reserved.
Library of Congress Cataloging-in-Publication is on file.
Library of Congress Control Number: 2023903330

ISBN: 978-1-7329132-5-7

This paperback original is published by
Sex Ed Talk LLC Omaha, NE
www.sexedtalk.com

1st Edition

Cover Design by Sara M. Lyons
Graphic Design by Carol Sayers
Book Layout by Michael Campbell, MC Writing Services

COLORS
of
YOU

Lesson Plans for Teachers and Parents
about Sex Education and Identity

• • •

Kristen Lilla LCSW, CST-S, CSE-S
and co-author
Christian Hoeger MA, MEd, LMHP

To our AMAB children, Aden, Christian, and Wilson

and to the kids at Girls Inc. of Omaha,
thank you for letting us teach you
and for teaching us

• • •

CONTENTS

PREFACE

It all started in 2013, when we met as co-workers at Girls Inc. of Omaha. We are both parents and therapists, but also have a passion for education, specifically sex education. Kristen (she/they) is a queer, Type-A workaholic who adores traveling, cats, and shoes. Christian (she/her) is an extroverted, laid-back woman who finds adventure traveling, eating at local spots, and scuba diving. Opposites in many ways, we are both opinionated, passionate, and boisterous, and it turns out we make a really great team!

Over the years we have collaborated on many projects. Our pride and joy is the publication of *Vaginas and Periods 101: A Pop-Up Book*. What started as a joke became a dream and then a reality in 2019. It is a fun and approachable way to teach menstruation, a classroom lesson plan we turned into a book. This innovative book has been sold worldwide. The pop-up book doesn't use pronouns or gender, keeping it inclusive for all.

After much success with the pop-up book, we wanted to create another accessible way to share the lesson plans we've developed and successfully used. We have so many ideas and have decided to put them all in one place: here! Most sex education books are focused on teenagers or college students, but after years of experience we know that everyone, even children, has a right to sex education that validates and responds to their curiosity and desire to learn.

Teaching over the years also made it evident that sex education isn't just about anatomy. Sexuality is about your feelings, your body, how you communicate, your gender, and more. The lessons throughout this book encapsulate these themes and more. Let's explore the colors of you...

INTRODUCTION FOR EDUCATORS

Discussing sex education with elementary age youth is an exciting privilege, but it can also be difficult. Many educators are not sure where to start the discussion, or if they are allowed to have the discussion at all. Questions start to loom: *is it appropriate? How will it make parents feel? How will the participants feel? How will it make me feel as an educator?* First, it is important to understand that sexuality encompasses everything from body image to anatomy to healthy communication. This acknowledgment helps offer educators and parents alike a place to start teaching sex education. Suddenly, sex education does not have to be overwhelming for you or the youth you teach. In fact, teaching this subject can be fun.

This manual offers hands-on lessons that can be implemented in just 45 minutes. The manual also offers assurance that each lesson was curated by professional sex educators and mental health professionals who have worked with youth for many years and have implemented these same lesson plans.

To make teaching this manual more comfortable for you, start by setting ground rules and expectations for both yourself and participants. Allow participants to help establish the ground rules for the classroom. Suggested ground rules include being respectful, permission to ask questions, permission to laugh, refraining from judgment, and encouraging participants to have further discussions about the handouts at home with their trusted adults. These simple but important guidelines help establish boundaries and will make the environment more comfortable for everyone.

Observe how your classroom is set up. Rearrange as needed, to create the best learning environment for your participants. It is important for participants to be comfortable in their environment. You could consider having everyone sit at a desk, moving the chairs into a circle, or having the participants sit on the floor. The arrangement may vary based on accessibility and lesson topic.

Be prepared that there may be times when an educator is put into an uncomfortable or awkward position. Perhaps a participant overshares or asks a question you don't have the answer to. What should you do when this happens? It is always an option to redirect the participant. Here are some things you might say:

- Thank you so much for sharing.
- I appreciate everyone sharing, but in the interest of time, we have to keep going.
- I'd love to talk with you more about this after class.
- What a great question. I don't know the answer, but I will look into it.
- I don't know.
- Great question. Why do you want to know that?
- Thanks for asking, but I don't want to make this about me.

You are embarking on a great adventure by implementing these lesson plans. The content and discussions that ensue can help provide increased self-esteem, acceptance, understanding, and growth for both you and the participants.

INTRODUCTION FOR TRUSTED ADULTS

We are so glad you picked up *Colors of You!* While these lesson plans are for youth, this manual is for you too! Having discussions with your child about sex education establishes trust, rapport, and bonding. The lessons throughout this manual are meant to be engaging and offer hands-on exercises so you can pursue what may feel like difficult conversations with direction and purpose. While the book is intended for educators, each lesson offers modifications so trusted adults, like parents and guardians, can implement the lessons outside of the classroom. Feel free to skip around and do the lessons in any order you want so they fit the conversations you are having at home.

•   •   •

The Body

"When children understand their bodies, the diversity of others, and learn how to set and respect boundaries, they stay safer, informed and more confident along the journey."

SEX POSITIVE FAMILIES, MELISSA CARNAGEY, LBSW

Throughout this section, participants will learn about their bodies, anatomy, how babies are made, and body hygiene. In order for children to experience autonomy and set boundaries, they need to be empowered to feel comfortable in their own skin by having the right language to advocate for themselves. Each lesson will help children learn more about their growing bodies in a way that feels fun and approachable.

• • •

LESSON 1:
This is My Body

Rationale:

Everyone has a body. Almost all of the body parts we possess, regardless of sex, are the same. Yet our bodies also all look different. This lesson plan will normalize the body and help participants understand basic anatomy.

Objectives:

- To identify which body parts we all have
- To develop skills and comfort in naming body parts

Modification for Parents/Guardians:

Instead of using the handout, parents may choose to have their child point to their own bodies to identify body parts. For example, you could say, "Show me where your arm is" and have your child point to their arm.

Materials:

- Chart paper
- Crayons
- Lesson 1 Handout on page 5

Lesson Plan:

1. Start by asking the group to make a list of their body parts. List them on the chart paper. Be sure to include all responses.

2. Provide each person with the handout and crayons. Ask them to write the correct body part name on the line next to that body part. If participants need help spelling the words correctly, you can offer assistance. Tell the

4 · COLORS *of* YOU

participants what a great job they did identifying different body parts on the body.

3. Have the group stand up. Tell them they will play a game called Simon Says. Explain that you will be Simon. Instruct the participants to follow your directions whenever you say, "Simon Says" followed by a directive. Tell the group if you just give a directive without saying "Simon Says," they will be asked to sit down and this will end their participation in the game. Be sure to include identifying body parts as you engage in game play, such as "Simon Says touch your arm." "Shake your leg." "Wiggle your hips." You may engage in several rounds of game play. You may opt to have the winner of the first round be "Simon" in the following round. If you want to, offer a small prize to the winner(s).

4. Congratulate the group on being able to identify so many of their body parts!

Opinion Questions:

- What body parts can we see?
- Can you name body parts that are not visible?
- What body parts do other animals have that are the same as us?
- What body parts do other animals have that are different from us?

Lesson 1 Handout

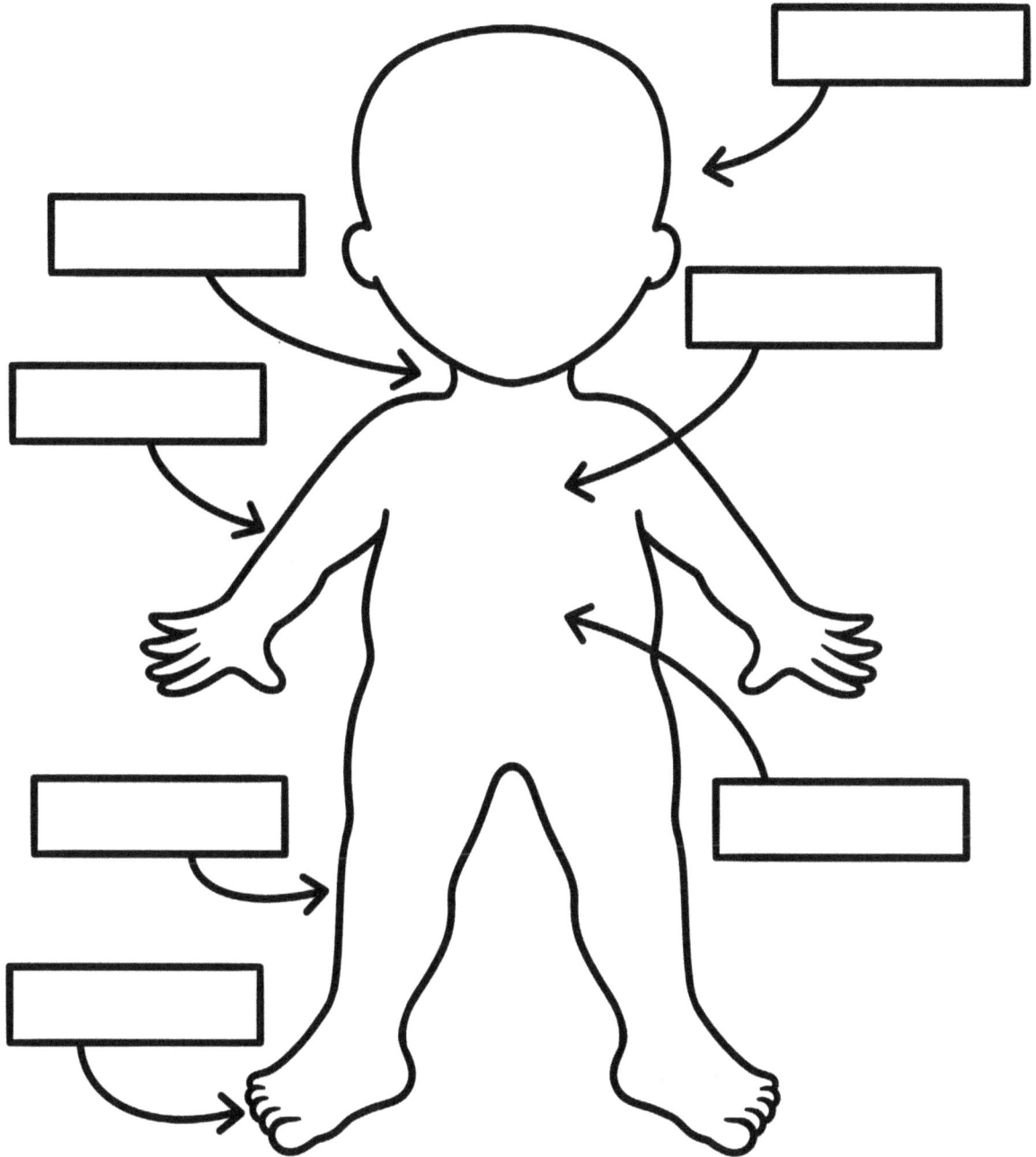

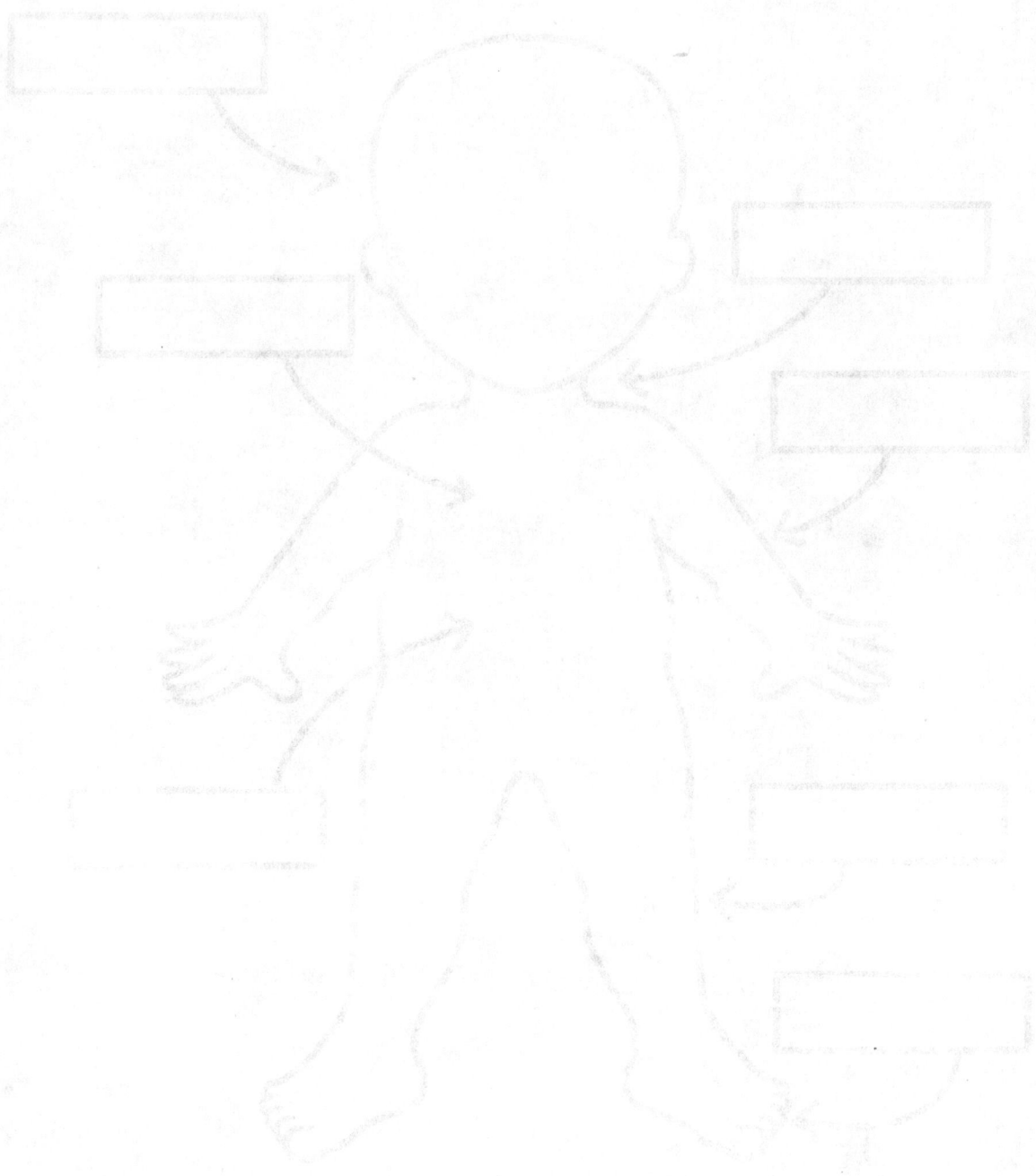

LESSON 2:
My Anatomy

Rationale:

Children who can accurately define and identify their genitals are less prone to be victims of sexual assault. Using incorrect terms or nicknames limits communication, reinforcing the idea that genitals are secret, and helping perpetrators maintain a victim's silence. While using the words "penis" or "vulva" can be embarrassing for adults, especially when the words are used in public, it serves as an opportunity to talk about privacy. Just as genitals are considered a private body part, talking about them is also a private conversation.

Normalizing anatomy is the consensus among sex education professionals and is endorsed by both The National Sexual Violence Resource Center and the American Academy of Pediatrics. A 2021 literature review of three decades of research found "strong evidence for the effectiveness of child sex abuse prevention efforts in elementary school" when school-based sex education is taught (Goldfarb, 2021).

Objectives:

- To identify and define the vulva and uterus
- To identify and define the testicles and penis

Modification for Parents/Guardians:

Trusted adults can use this lesson as an opportunity to correctly define genitalia and normalize anatomy. It is also an opportunity for trusted adults to have a discussion with their child about privacy. Trusted adults can normalize children touching their genitals while stressing the importance of doing it only in private, such as in the bathroom or bedroom. Trusted adults can also use this opportunity to discuss that it is okay to touch our own genitals, but not for someone else to do so, unless it is a parent, guardian, or doctor, and they are doing so with the child's permission. This can also be an opportunity to reinforce that discussing genitals is a private conversation that is okay to have with trusted adults, but not in public or at school.

Materials:

- Lesson 2 Handouts on page 11

Lesson Plan:

1. Ask participants to recall the last lesson, when they identified a variety of body parts all people have. Explain that in this lesson, you will discuss body parts that can make people different from one another.

2. Explain to the participants that some of the body parts that will be discussed are visible and some are not, just like our arms are visible but our heart is inside of our bodies. Acknowledge there may be some initial embarrassment and giggles. The handouts are pictures showing the parts of our body that we consider private. Since they are considered private, we keep them covered by our clothes, except at bath time, going to the bathroom or changing, or at the doctor's office.

3. Provide each participant with the two handouts. Ask if anyone knows what they are looking at. Congratulate anyone who is able to identify the uterus, vulva, testicles, or penis.

4. Have participants look at the handout of the vulva and uterus. Explain that the vulva is a body part some people have. The vulva is what may be seen when those people go to the bathroom. Then explain that people born with vulvas also have a uterus. The uterus is located inside the body, and is the squishy middle part below the belly button. Have everyone squish their tummy below their belly button. Explain that they cannot feel it because it is inside the body, just like our hearts. Tell the participants that inside the uterus is where babies grow.

5. Have participants look at the handout of the scrotum and penis. Explain that the scrotum and penis are body parts that some people have. People with a penis use this body part to urinate when they go to the bathroom. Explain

that below the penis is the scrotum, which contains the testicles. The testicles are a body part that helps make babies.

6. It is important to explain to participants that each of our genitals looks different on different people, just like our noses. Introduce participants to the word "intersex." The Intersex Society of North America states, "Intersex is a general term used for a variety of conditions in which a person is born with a reproductive or sexual anatomy that doesn't seem to fit the typical definitions of female or male." Explain that some people are born with genitals that don't quite look like the ones in the handouts and may be intersex. Their anatomy might look different on the outside or on the inside, so they might not even know they are intersex, but they are still normal and healthy people.

7. Allow the participants to giggle and ask questions. Answer their questions honestly and accurately. If you do not know an answer to a question, it is okay to say this. If a question makes you uncomfortable, direct the child to talk to their trusted adult.

Opinion Questions:

- Did you know any of these terms before today?

- What do you call your private parts or genitals? What words do your trusted adults use?

- How does saying these words make you feel? What about the new words you learned?

Lesson 2 Handouts

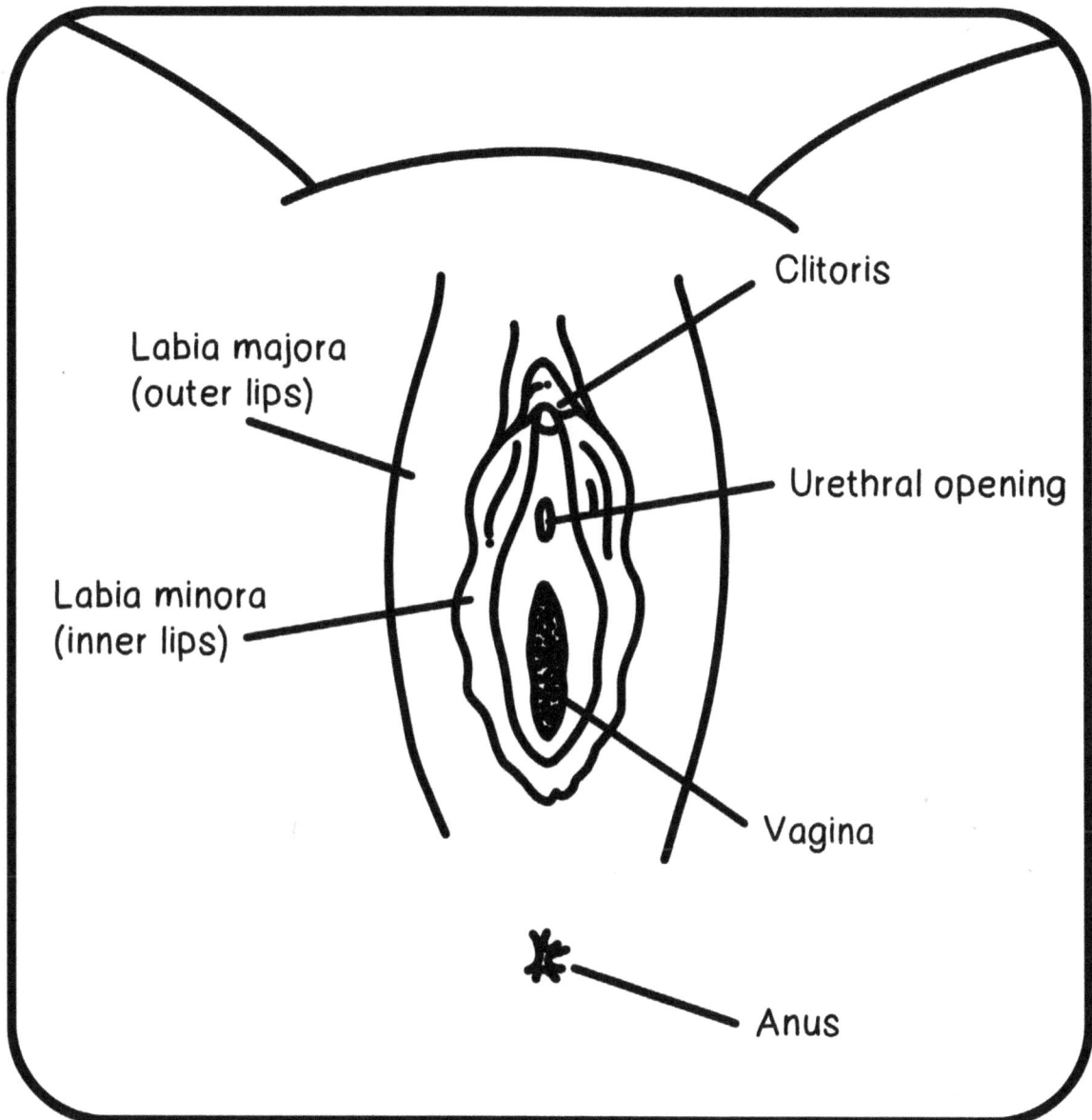

Clitoris

Labia majora
(outer lips)

Urethral opening

Labia minora
(inner lips)

Vagina

Anus

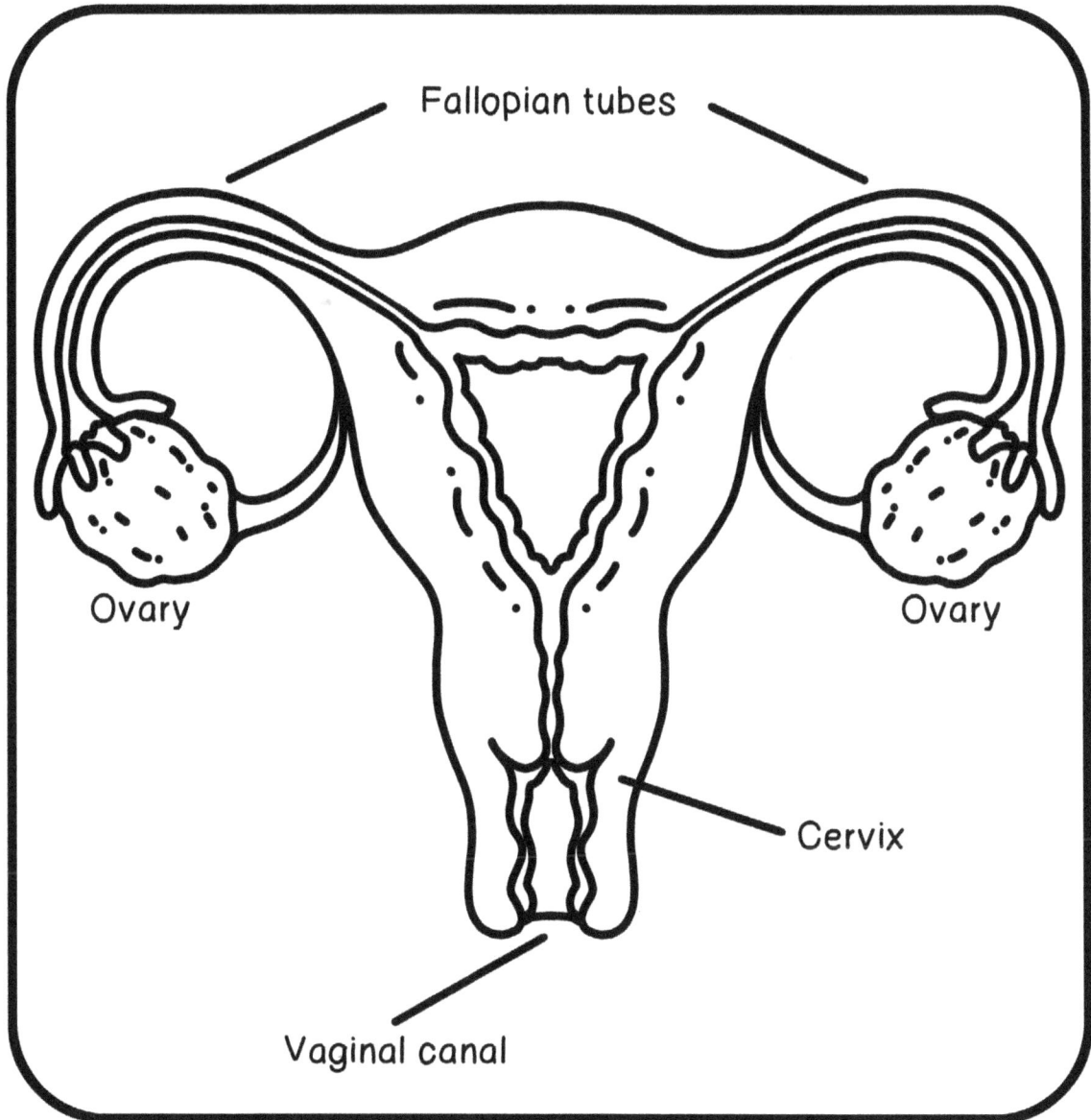

Fallopian tubes

Ovary

Ovary

Cervix

Vaginal canal

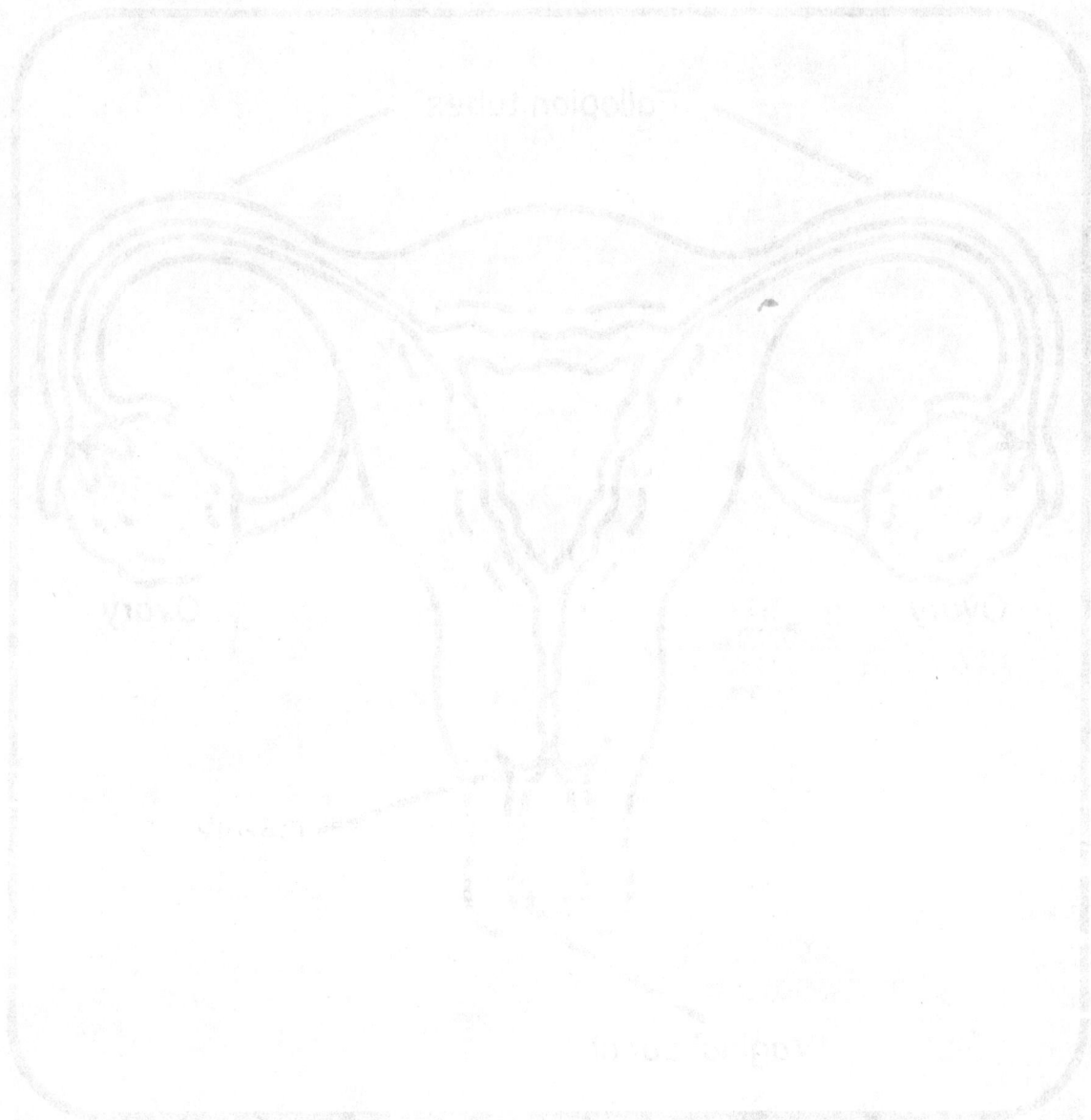

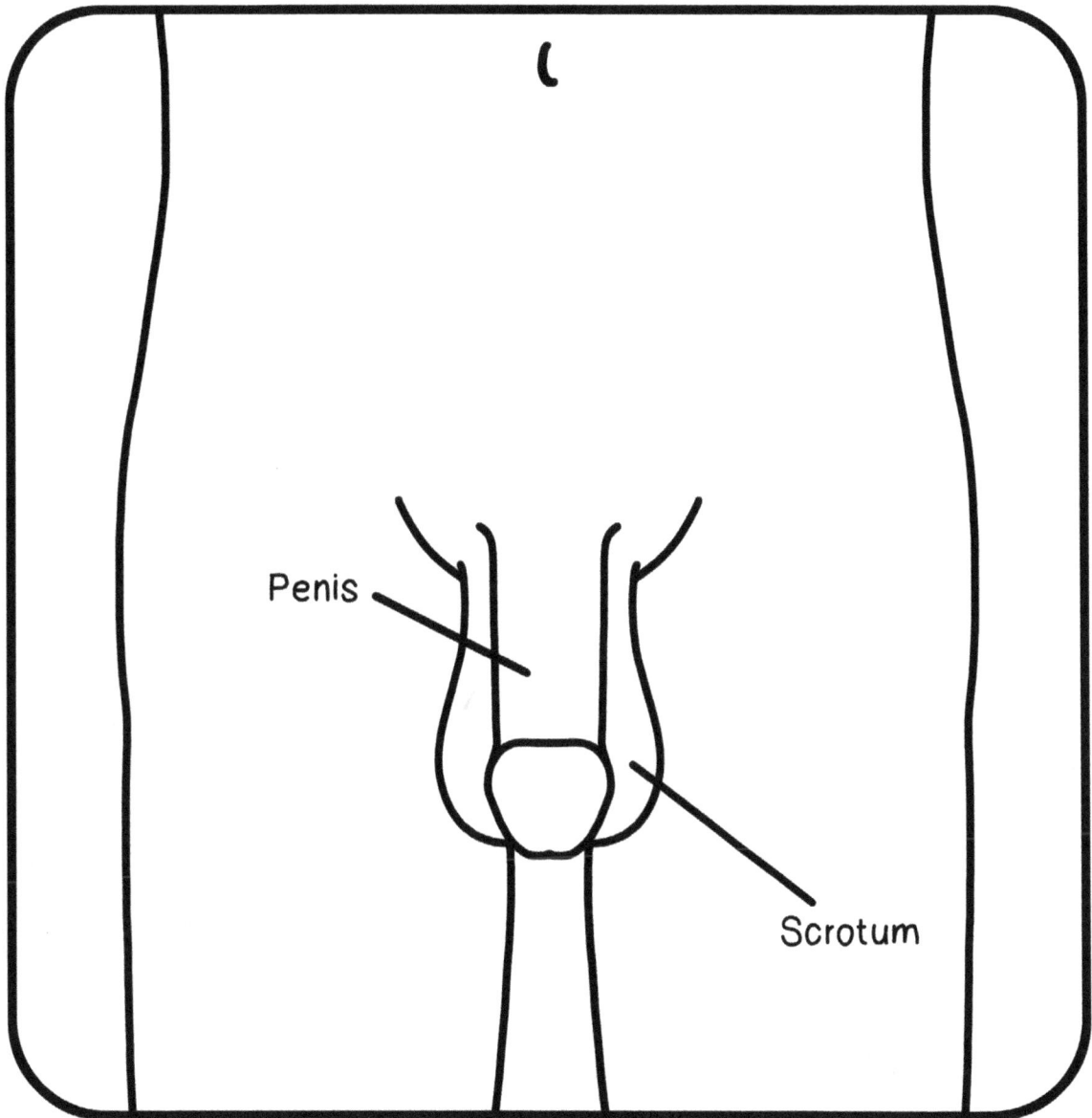

Penis

Scrotum

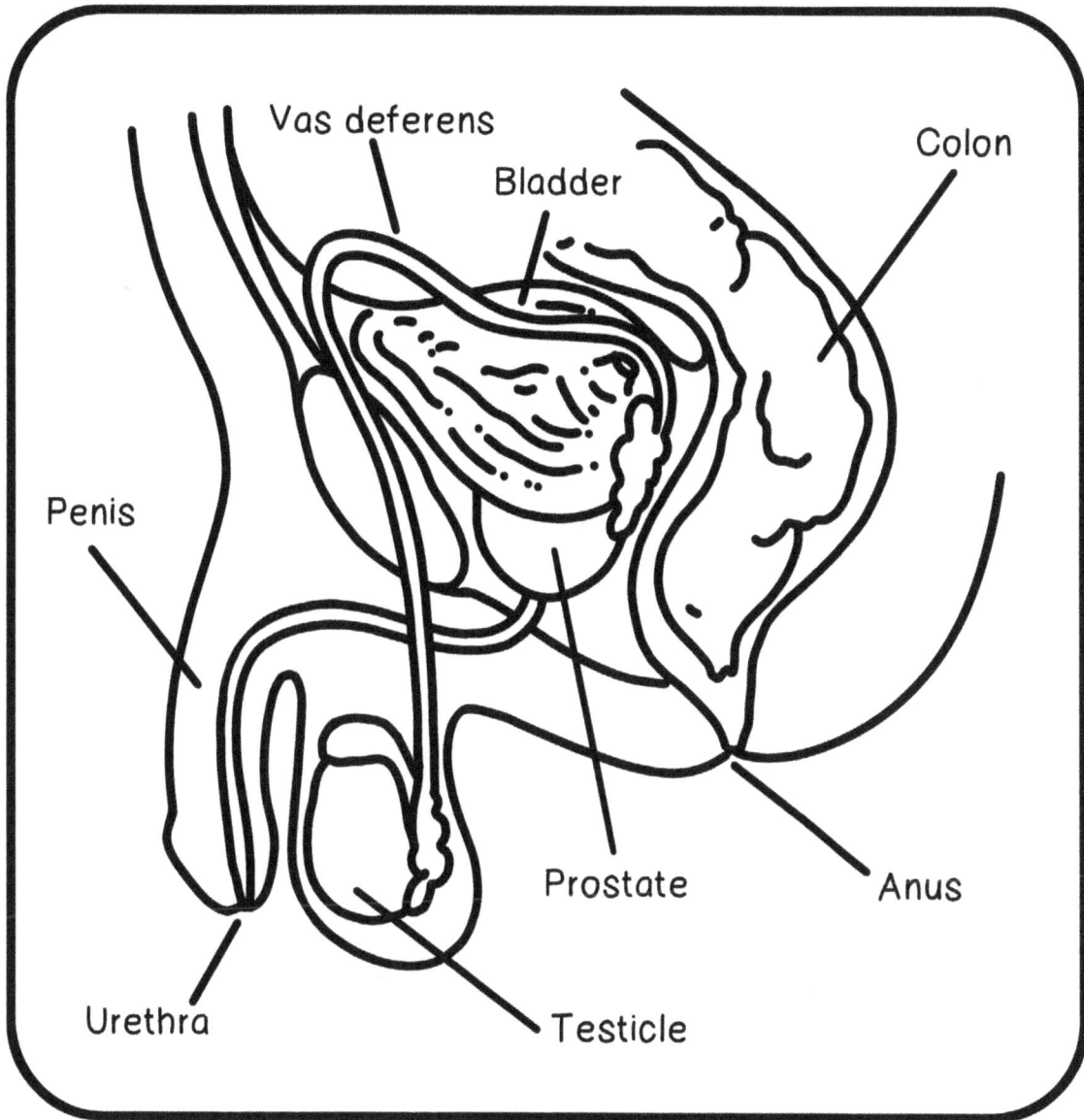

Vas deferens

Colon

Bladder

Penis

Prostate

Anus

Urethra

Testicle

LESSON 3:
Where Did I Come From?

Rationale:

The goal of this lesson is for youth to understand physiologically how a baby is made. They will learn about the reproductive organs some people have and that cells in the body—sperm and egg cells—enable people to reproduce when they unite. The information provided in this lesson is medically accurate. It will also provide youth with an opportunity to ask questions about their own bodies, how babies are made, as well as offer further understanding of reproduction and anatomy. This lesson was created to be inclusive of children who have been adopted, conceived via IVF, or are in foster care. Please utilize the previous lesson, My Anatomy, to identify body parts and establish shared vocabulary.

Objectives:

- Explain that some people have sperm
- Explain that some people have eggs
- Explain that a sperm and an egg come together to make a baby

Modification for Parents/Guardians:

Trusted adults, you may choose to personalize this lesson with your child by sharing the story of how they were conceived: about the pregnancy, where they were born, and who was there to meet them for the first time.

Materials:

- Chart paper
- Red crayons
- Blue crayons
- Yellow crayons
- 8½ by 11½" cardstock
- Hair dryer
- Glue
- Optional book: *What Makes a Baby* by Cory Silverberg

Lesson Plan:

1. Explain to participants they are going to learn how babies are made and where they come from. Establish ground rules for the group to follow such as encouraging questions, permission to laugh, being respectful, and "to put on our science hats."

2. Post a piece of chart paper labeled, "How Babies Are Made." Ask the participants, "How do you think babies are made?" Record their responses on the chart paper.

3. On another piece of chart paper, write, "Where Babies Come From." Ask the participants, "Where do you think babies come from?" Record their responses on the chart paper.

4. Remind the class what was discussed in Lesson #2 and review genital anatomy.

5. Provide each participant with handouts from Lesson #2 and discuss the following points:

   - Some people have sperm, and some people have eggs.
   - When a sperm and an egg come together, they create something new, a science word called a zygote. A zygote is a bundle of cells, shaped like a ball. A zygote is so small you cannot even see it with your eyes. It is even smaller than the period at the end of a sentence!
   - The zygote attaches to the uterus, which is inside the body below the belly button.

- The zygote grows and grows until it becomes a baby. It grows for nine months.
- When the baby is ready to come out, the uterus helps push the baby out through the vaginal canal.
- Babies may be born at the hospital, at home, or at a birthing center. Babies are cute but require a lot of attention!

6. Ask participants if they have any questions. Repeat Step Four if necessary. This is also when you can read the optional book *What Makes a Baby* by Cory Silverberg.

7. To learn how two things become one, the participants will now do an activity. Each child will need two different colored crayons and a piece of cardstock. Have them write their names on one side of the cardstock. On the other side, glue the two different colored crayons on the paper so they stay in place. Be sure to remove the wrapper before gluing. Then, with an adult's help, plug in the hairdryer and hold it up to the crayons. As the crayons melt together, they will blend to create a new color. Lay the pictures down so the melted crayons can dry on the cardstock. After each child has had an opportunity to melt their crayons on the cardstock, have them sit back down to engage in the questions that follow.

Opinion Questions:

- What did melting two crayons together do?
- How is a baby made?
- Why do we need two things to create something new?
- When is your birthday?
- Where were you born?
- Do you have siblings with the same parents as you? Do you look alike?
- Do you look like your parents?

LESSON 4:
Getting Clean from Head to Toe

Rationale:

Staying clean is important at any age to maintain health and fight off illness and infection. Bathing is essential to remove dirt and bacteria from our bodies. It keeps us smelling fresh and clean too. This becomes more important as we hit puberty and develop sweat glands. Teaching about personal hygiene is essential so participants can learn about cleanliness and bodily autonomy. It should be noted that bathing requirements do vary based on culture and religion.

Objectives:

- To explain the importance of hygiene and bathing
- To illustrate ways to engage in personal hygiene

Modification for Parents/Guardians:

This is an opportunity to talk to your child about expectations regarding bathing and cleanliness at your home. You could personalize this lesson by discussing what you use as part of your personal routine. You might also choose to engage your child by taking them to the store and allowing them to select their own bath products.

Materials:

- Chart paper
- Marker

- Spatula and whisk
- Two bowls
- 1 cup of baking soda
- ¼ cup of cream of tartar
- ½ cup of cornstarch
- ½ cup of salt (Epsom salt or sea salt)
- 2 teaspoons of essential oil (example: tea tree oil, witch-hazel, lavender)
- 1 tablespoon of coconut oil
- Silicone ice cube tray
- Water
- Optional: food coloring

You may need additional ingredients based on the number of participants in your class. The above ingredients will make approximately 24 bath bombs.

Lesson Plan:

1. Start by asking the group to make a list of ways they keep their bodies clean. Use a marker to list them on the chart paper. Be sure to include all responses. Tell the participants that staying clean is something called "personal hygiene." Elaborate that personal hygiene consists of many of the items they listed and includes brushing teeth, combing hair, taking a bath/shower, putting on deodorant, and washing our hands.

2. Ask the participants, "Is it important to have personal hygiene?" Elicit all responses from participants. Explain to participants the need for better hygiene as they age. Be sure to explain that it is important to wash the areas where we sweat the most, including our face, armpits, hands, and feet.

3. Tell the participants that, to help promote personal hygiene, they will be making their own bath bombs. Bath bombs can be used as part of a bathing routine in the tub and will help them get clean, just like soap.

4. Put all the dry ingredients together in a bowl: baking soda, cream of tartar, cornstarch, and salt. Mix with a whisk. To save time, you may choose to have this step completed before beginning the lesson, depending on classroom size and set-up.

5. In another bowl, mix the wet ingredients with a spatula: essential oil, coconut oil, and optional food coloring.

6. Pour the wet ingredients into the bowl with the dry ingredients. Mix the ingredients together with a spatula or whisk. Add water as needed so the ingredients blend together until the texture is similar to wet sand.

7. Once the mixture sticks together like wet sand, divide the substance into the ice cube tray. Pack the mixture into each cube. Let it sit overnight to solidify. Note that the mixture will expand. Each cube is now a bath bomb. Give each participant a bath bomb to take home. Instruct them to fill the tub with warm water and put the bath bomb into the water. It will fizz in the water and help them get clean.

8. As a classroom, clean up together, and then answer the opinion questions as a group.

Opinion Questions:

- What did you learn from today's lesson about personal hygiene and cleanliness?

- What makes getting clean fun?

- How can you encourage your friends or siblings to take care of their personal hygiene?

- What other ideas do you have about staying clean?

LESSON 5:
What is Sex?

Rationale:

At an early age, kids begin asking questions about where babies came from and how they are made. Adults are often unwilling to answer the question or end up providing inaccurate responses. This can be confusing for children who are trying to understand their bodies and build trusting relationships with adults. This lesson provides the skills you need to discuss with children the basics of how babies are made. Helping children know the definition of sex will make it more likely they will tell a trusted adult if they are ever assaulted. Note that this lesson can be taught before/after/with Lesson #3. If you decide to proceed with the lesson, and children have additional questions, you should instruct them to talk to their trusted adults. You may also choose to make this a parent-child event.

If you are doing this in a classroom setting, it is advised to send home a permission slip before doing this lesson. Find the sample Sex Education Permission Slip on page 127.

Objectives:

- To define the act of sex

Modification for Parents/Guardians:

If children are asking questions about sex, it is okay to answer them. Do not feel obligated to offer a detailed response but do be sure to answer their questions honestly. This lesson is an opportunity to become a trusted adult and resource for your child.

Materials:

- Lesson 5 Handout on page 29

Lesson Plan:

Use the handout provided. The handout provides a guided script for talking to children about sex and childbirth. It also provides resources for adults and children to continue conversations about sexuality. You may choose to share all of the information in the handout, or just some of it. After you have read through the script, ask the following opinion questions.

Opinion Questions:

- Do you understand what the act of sex means?
- How does it feel to know what the act of sex is?
- Do you understand why kids cannot have sex?
- Do you have questions about what it means to consent?
- Who would you talk to if someone tried to touch you without your permission?
- What other questions do you have?

Additional Resources for Adults:

- *From Diapers to Dating: A Parent's Guide to Raising Sexually Healthy Children – From Infancy to Middle School* by Reverend Debra Haffner
- *Talk to Me First: Everything You Need to Know to Become Your Kids' "Go-To" Person about Sex* by Deborah Roffman
- *Read Me: A Parental Primer for "The Talk"* by Lanae St. John
- *Breaking the Hush Factor: Ten Rules for Talking with Teens* by Dr. Karen Rayne, PhD

Additional Resources for Kids:

- *The Science of Babies* by Deborah Roffman
- *Sex is a Funny Word* by Cory Silverberg

Lesson 5 Handout

What is Sex?

Sex is an act that occurs between people, usually adults. Oftentimes, it is a way for two people who love each other to express their love. Sometimes adults have sex just because it feels good. Men and women may have sex. Women may have sex with other women and men may have sex with other men. Before people have sex, they get naked so their bodies can be close to one another, and their skin can touch.

Sex can happen in several ways. One common way for two people to have sex is when a penis goes inside a vagina. Without preventative steps, this is how babies are made. (You may choose to reference Lesson #3.) Two people may also have sex when one person puts their mouth on the other person's penis or vagina. This is called oral sex. It can be pleasurable for adults but does not result in making a baby. People may also insert a penis into the anus (butthole). This is called anal sex. This also does not make a baby. Adults may choose to do all of these different kinds of sex, or none of them at all.

One thing that is very important to know about sex is that it should be between people who *consent*. This means both people know what they are agreeing to and want to be doing it. Kids cannot consent to sex, because their bodies are not big enough to understand having sex in a safe and consensual way. A kid should never have sex with an adult, and an adult should never ask a kid to have sex. If this ever happens, say no, and tell someone right away. Do not keep it as a secret.

There are ways kids and adults can show each other they love each other which are appropriate, including a high-five, holding hands, and hugs. (Please refer to Lesson #11 for additional discussion and examples.)

Identity

"We are not what other people say we are. We are who we know ourselves to be, and we are what we love. That's okay."

LAVERNE COX

"Loving other people starts with loving ourselves and accepting ourselves."

ELLIOT PAGE

Feeling confident in who we are is affirming. Expressing who we are is freeing. Understanding why we are special is empowering. This section does all of these and more as it explores gender roles, gender expression, body image, uniqueness, and self-esteem. All of these areas of identity are important components for an individual to develop a healthy identity now and into adulthood. Developing an earlier sense of identity and confidence leads to healthier relationships and eventual understanding of one's sexuality.

• • •

LESSON 6:
Boys Can, Girls Can

Rationale:

"Studies suggest that most children develop the ability to label gender groups and to use gender labels in their speech between 18 and 24 months," share Martin and Ruble in their research titled *Patterns of Gender and Development*. Despite being so young, Martin and Ruble found these labels and "knowing basic gender information was related to increased play with strongly stereotyped toys." Gender stereotypes can negatively affect children and limit their interests to traditional gender roles. By creating gender diversity and exposing stereotypes rather than limiting gender roles, children are empowered to engage in more activities and opportunities they enjoy.

Objectives:

- To describe how gender roles and gender stereotypes affect us

Modification for Parents/Guardians:

Discuss with your child the gender roles you take on. Also discuss how you defy gender roles and stereotypes. Ask your children how they feel about gender roles and stereotypes. This will help assess the need for continued conversation. There are also many books you can read with your child about breaking gender stereotypes. Find one that resonates with you and your family. Suggested titles include *Is That For a Boy or a Girl?* by S. Bear Bergman and *Jacob's New Dress* by Sarah Hoffman.

Materials:

- Chart paper
- Markers
- Stickers

Lesson Plan:

1. Greet the class. Tell them they will be talking about how boys and girls are perceived as similar and different.

2. Get two pieces of chart paper to hang. On one piece of chart paper, draw a box and label the chart **GIRLS**. On the second piece of chart paper, draw a box and label the chart **BOYS**.

3. Ask the participants to brainstorm, or think of things that girls like to do. Write their responses in the box that says GIRLS.

4. Ask the participants to brainstorm, or think of things that boys like to do. Write their responses in the box that says BOYS.

5. Pointing to the sheet labeled GIRLS, ask the participants, "Are there things in the box boys can do too?" Put a sticker next to the ones the class says boys can do too. Most, if not all, should have a sticker.

6. Using the sheet labeled BOYS, ask the participants, "Are there things in the box girls can do too?" Put a sticker next to the ones the class says girls can do too. Most, if not all, should have a sticker.

7. When they say only a girl can do things, or only a boy can do things, tell the class this is called a gender stereotype. Elaborate that gender stereotypes are assumptions we make about people because of their gender or how they look. Continue to the opinion questions.

Opinion Questions:

- What are the things you like to do that are considered a gender stereotype? Offer an example if you need to. For example, "only girls can dance ballet" and "only boys can play football."

- What are the things you like to do that break gender stereotypes? Offer an example if you need to. For example, "as a girl I enjoy playing basketball" and "as a boy I enjoy painting my nails."

- Do you think it is fair to put people into these boxes or limit someone's activities to what is in these boxes? How might this affect someone? (This could also be an opportunity to talk about non-binary or transgender youth.)

LESSON 7:
The Gender Expression Trunk

Rationale:

Gender expression is how a person expresses themselves through their clothing and mannerisms. It is the way people present themselves to the world and, as a form of expression, it is a visible way to present to others how they want to be seen. Gender expression evolves and changes over time and varies throughout cultures. Discussing the concept of gender expression allows children to be comfortable with how they express themselves.

Objectives:

- To define gender expression
- To illustrate gender expression

Modification for Parents/Guardians:

This is an opportunity to encourage children to express themselves in a way that feels comfortable for them. Share how you express your gender through your clothes and dress. There are many books where children express themselves in ways beyond the binary, including *Oliver Button is a Sissy* by Tomie DePaola and *The Paper Bag Princess* by Robert Munsch.

Materials:

- Trunk (or a box decorated like a trunk)
- Variety of dress-up clothes

- Note: If no dress-up clothes are available, consider having students draw pictures or use magazine cut-outs to create an outfit. Students can also use brown paper bags to make clothes.

Lesson Plan:

1. Start the lesson by welcoming the class. Then ask the participants, "Why did you choose to put on the outfit you are wearing today?" Encourage all responses. Share why you chose to wear the outfit you are wearing today.

2. Ask the participants, "Did any of you do your own hair today? Or pick out your own hair accessories? Did anyone decide to wear a hat today? What shoes did you decide to wear today?" Have volunteers share why they styled their hair a certain way or picked out the accessories they are wearing.

3. Point out to the class that it is fun to express ourselves through our clothing and how we do our hair. Tell the class the way they share themselves with the world is called gender expression. If you did Lesson #6, remind them that boys and girls are often told to dress or act a certain way, and do specific activities. Remind them this is called a gender stereotype. Provide a stereotype for the class. For example, "girls do ballet" and "boys play basketball." Ask, "can boys also do ballet and can girls also play basketball?" When they say yes, tell the class the same is true of wearing outfits. Clothes are just fabric we wear. Boys and girls can wear any clothes they feel comfortable in.

4. Consider showing the class pictures of different gender expressions across a variety of cultures worldwide. Examples might include outfits and traditional wear from Western culture, African tribes, Islamic culture, Rabari, Scottish kilts, and more.

5. Tell the participants they will have an opportunity to share their own gender expression now. You can inform them you have a whole trunk full of clothes and you want them to pick out a piece of clothing that speaks to them, or inspires them, and seems fun or comfortable. You may also tell the class they will be making their own clothing if you choose to use magazines and paper bags to create outfits.

6. Once participants have chosen something to wear, have them show the class their outfit. You can make it a fashion show if you have the space to do so.

7. After everyone has had an opportunity to select an outfit from the trunk, or make an outfit and show the class, have them sit back down in a circle and engage in the following opinion questions.

Opinion Questions:

- Can someone remind us what gender expression is?
- What is fun about expressing yourself through your clothing and hairstyle?
- Is there anything not fun about it? How come?
- What influences you to wear certain colors or styles of clothing?
- How do you feel about girls who wear pants?
- How do you feel about boys who wear dresses? (Address any negative responses in a way that is supportive of anyone wearing what they want to.)

LESSON 8:
My Positive Body Image

Rationale:

How we view our bodies affects both our confidence and self-esteem. Children begin to understand the concept of body image between ages 2 and 5. According to a study by Common Sense Media, 25% of kids have attempted a diet by the age of seven. Instilling positive messages about body image can help youth have a greater sense of self and bodily autonomy.

Objectives:

- To define body image
- To illustrate positive views of self and body image

Modification for Parents/Guardians:

Discuss with your child how you viewed yourself at their age. Show them a picture of you at that age if you have one. Share with them what you thought you would be doing when you grew up. Elaborate on how that has looked the same and how it has changed. Be sure to take part in the lesson plan with them, drawing a picture of you now and how you saw yourself as a child.

Materials:

- Crayons, colored pencils, or markers
- White paper
- Chart paper

Lesson Plan:

1. Ask participants if they can tell you what body image means. Give all participants an opportunity to respond and record their responses on chart paper.

2. Offer them the following definition of body image from the Office on Women's Health: "Your body image is what you think and how you feel when you look in the mirror or when you picture yourself in your mind. This includes how you feel about your appearance; what you think about your body itself, such as your height and weight; and how you feel within your own skin."

3. On chart paper, ask participants to list things that would encourage positive views of body image. Record their responses.

4. On another piece of chart paper, ask participants to list things that make a person have poor body image and record their responses.

5. On a fourth piece of chart paper, write "Influences" at the top. Ask participants *who* and *what* influence our views of body image. Be sure to include "media" in their responses.

6. Explain that a person's view of their body image also influences their self-esteem and confidence. Give each child a piece of white paper and coloring utensils. Tell the group they are going to draw a picture of how they see themselves now, and a second picture of how they see themselves as an adult.

7. Once the group has completed their drawings, discuss the following opinion questions and give participants an opportunity to share their drawings.

Opinion Questions:

- In the drawing of yourself now, do you have a positive or poor image of your body? Why? How can you tell? If you receive a response of "poor image," utilize some of the suggestions from the Influences chart to help the participant gain a positive image.

- In the picture you drew of yourself all grown up, do you have a positive or poor body image? Why? How can you tell?

- If you have positive views of your body, what might change to make it poor?

- If you see yourself having a poor body image, what might change to make it positive?

LESSON 9:
I'm a Unique Flower

Rationale:

Even with over 7 billion people in the world, we are all interested in different hobbies and activities, which make each of us unique. This lesson will focus on highlighting what makes each individual participant unique. Kids begin to feel peer pressure at a young age, which increases throughout adolescence, before it wanes again in adulthood. As participants begin to feel pressure to fit in with their peers, they tend to mirror their opinions and interests. Emphasizing that our unique individual qualities are what make us interesting will encourage participants to diversify.

Objectives:

- To define diversity
- To describe individual differences that make each of us unique
- To encourage participants to view their differences positively

Modification for Parents/Guardians:

Complete this activity with your child. Engaging in the activity will demonstrate your own uniqueness to your child, and give you an opportunity to discuss differences and similarities within your own family. Be sure to commend your child on what makes them special. You may choose to hang their artwork from this lesson to validate you are proud they are able to identify their unique qualities. If your family comes from a diverse background, be sure to share and discuss this information with your child.

Materials:

- Craft sticks

- Lesson 9 Handout on page 45, or construction paper
- Glue
- Markers
- Scissors
- Photograph of each child (printed or drawn)
- Chart paper

Lesson Plan:

1. Invite the participants to the lesson and tell them they are going to do a very special lesson today. Explain that it is special because not only is it about each one of them, but it is also about helping you make a unique and diverse garden.

2. Then, on a piece of chart paper, write the word "unique." Ask the participants if they know what the word means and invite responses. Thank them for their answers, and then confirm the word unique is used to describe the things that make us special and different from one another.

3. On another piece of chart paper, ask the participants to call out things that make them unique. They can list hobbies, personality traits, or physical features. Write down as many responses as you can and encourage each participant to contribute.

4. Explain that being unique and different also adds to diversity. Offer the following definition for diversity: being different.

5. Next, tell the participants they will create an art project to highlight what makes them special, unique, and diverse by creating a "Me Flower." Give each participant one popsicle stick, glue, markers, scissors, and construction paper or the handout. They will also need a photograph of themselves. If you are unable to obtain a photograph of each child, have them take a few minutes to draw a picture of themselves.

6. Participants will now construct their Me Flower.

   ◦ If the participants have the handout, tell them to use the scissors to cut out the petals and circle.
   ◦ If they have construction paper, first have the participants cut a circle for the center of the flower. Then instruct them to use the construction paper

to cut out petals. Participants should do a minimum of five petals and a maximum of ten petals.

7. Instruct participants to use the markers to write unique qualities that make them different on each of the petals. They can list hobbies, personality traits, or physical features. They can also refer back to the list they made earlier in the lesson for ideas.

8. Encourage the participants to glue their photograph or the drawing of themselves onto the circle. This is the center of their Me Flower.

9. Have participants glue the tips of the petals onto the circle. Be sure they glue the petals so the words and photograph are visible.

10. Last, have them glue the popsicle stick on to create the flower's stem. They may choose to color the popsicle stick or write their name on it.

11. Once participants have finished their art projects, ask the following questions and encourage them to share their Me Flowers. Display them in your classroom as a garden. To highlight and celebrate diversity, point out that gardens are prettiest when they are made up of many unique and diverse flowers.

Opinion Questions:

- What unique quality are you most proud of?
- Is there ever a time you have wanted to be like everyone else? When? Why?
- How do you imagine the petals will change over time? How will they stay the same?

Lesson 9 Handout

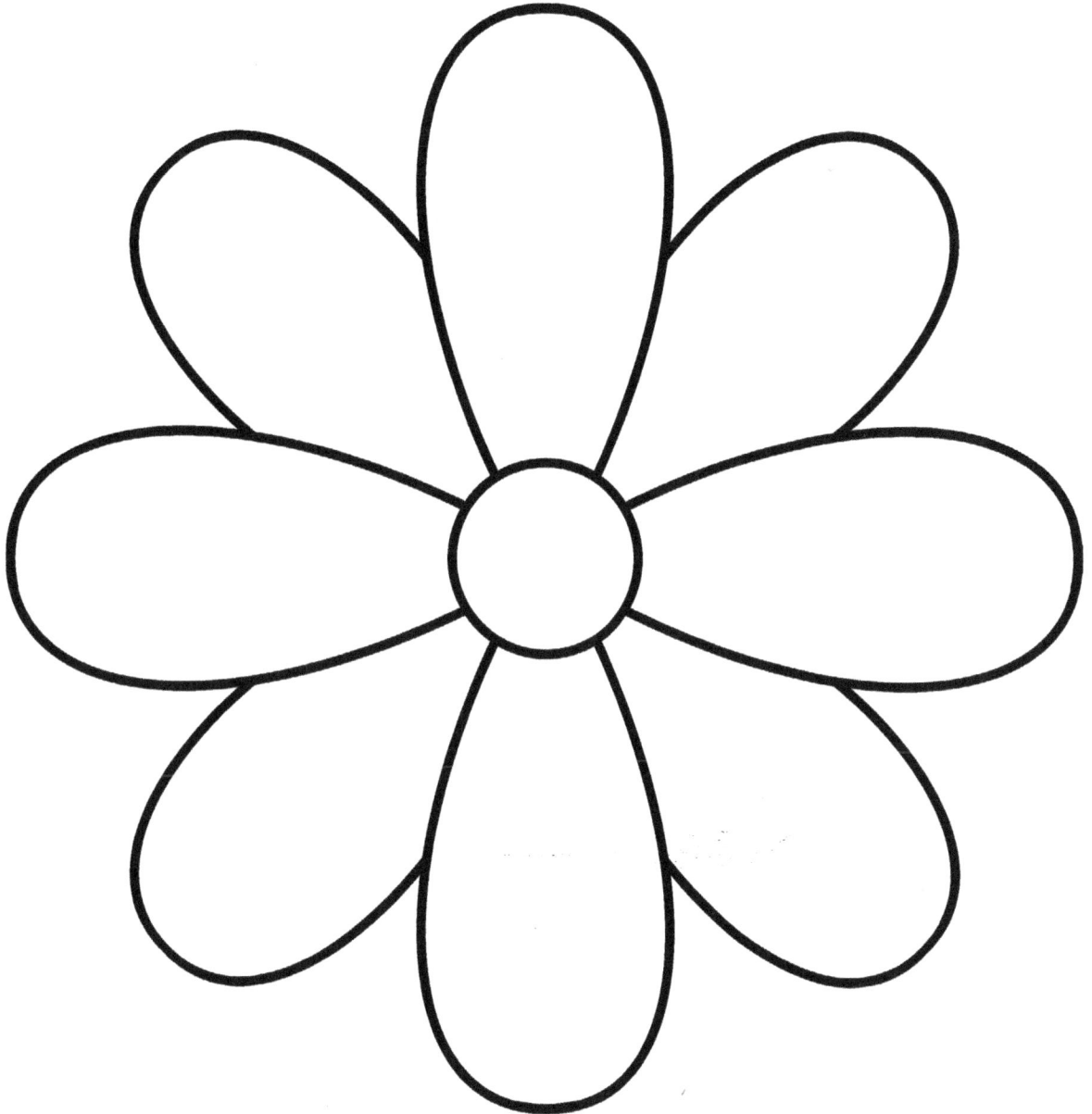

LESSON 10:
Feeling My Self (Esteem)

Rationale:

Creating self-esteem is an important piece of having confidence, a positive self-image, and self-assurance. Children with self-esteem are more likely to feel proud of themselves, try harder at new activities, believe in themselves, and advocate for themselves. Kids with low self-esteem may be self-critical, find it more difficult to deal with failure, and may be more likely to give up.

Objectives:

- To define self-esteem
- To illustrate ways to build self-esteem

Modification for Parents/Guardians:

Self-esteem often starts at home and is higher when children feel loved, cared for, and accepted. You can help build your child's self-esteem by telling them you are proud of them, giving them words of affirmation, encouraging them to try new activities, and focusing on their strengths. To modify the activity, you can encourage your child to write a card to themselves on an ongoing basis. You can also do the compliment game as a family activity.

Materials:

- Lesson 10 Handout on page 51, or construction paper
- Markers or crayons
- White paper

- Tape
- Scissors

Lesson Plan:

1. Since today's lesson is about building self-esteem, welcome the class by telling them how wonderful they are and how proud you are of their hard work.

2. Now ask them to share something they are proud of about themselves. After everyone has an opportunity to answer the question, congratulate them on having positive self-esteem. Elaborate: self-esteem is how we feel about ourselves, and having high self-esteem helps us feel proud and confident.

3. Tell the class they will now play a game. Each participant will need a piece of white paper. At the top of the paper have participants write their name. Then tape the paper onto each participant's back. Tell the class they will then walk around and write something they like about each participant on their back. Make sure each person writes on every participant's paper, so everyone is included in the activity. Give participants 10 minutes to do this activity.

4. When they finish, have them sit down and take the paper off of their back. Give each participant a few minutes to read over the compliments they received. Ask a few participants to share. Encourage students to hang these up at home to look at whenever they need a reminder of how awesome they are.

5. Next, they will do another art activity. There are two options: give each participant a copy of the printed heart handout, or have participants make their own heart using their favorite color of construction paper.

6. Tell participants the heart is to remind them they are each very special and loved. Next, instruct participants to write themselves a Valentine's Day letter that says how great they are. If it is not Valentine's Day, remind the class that it is important to know how special and loved they are every day. Encourage participants to decorate their Valentine's cards.

7. When everyone has finished, ask a few participants to share their cards, then move on to the opinion questions.

Opinion Questions:

- How did it feel walking around getting things written on your back?
- How did it feel when you got to read what was written on your back?
- How did it feel to write a Valentine's Day card to yourself?
- How did these activities increase your self-esteem?
- What are other things you do for your self-esteem?
- What are some things you can do to help others have more self-esteem?

Lesson 10 Handout

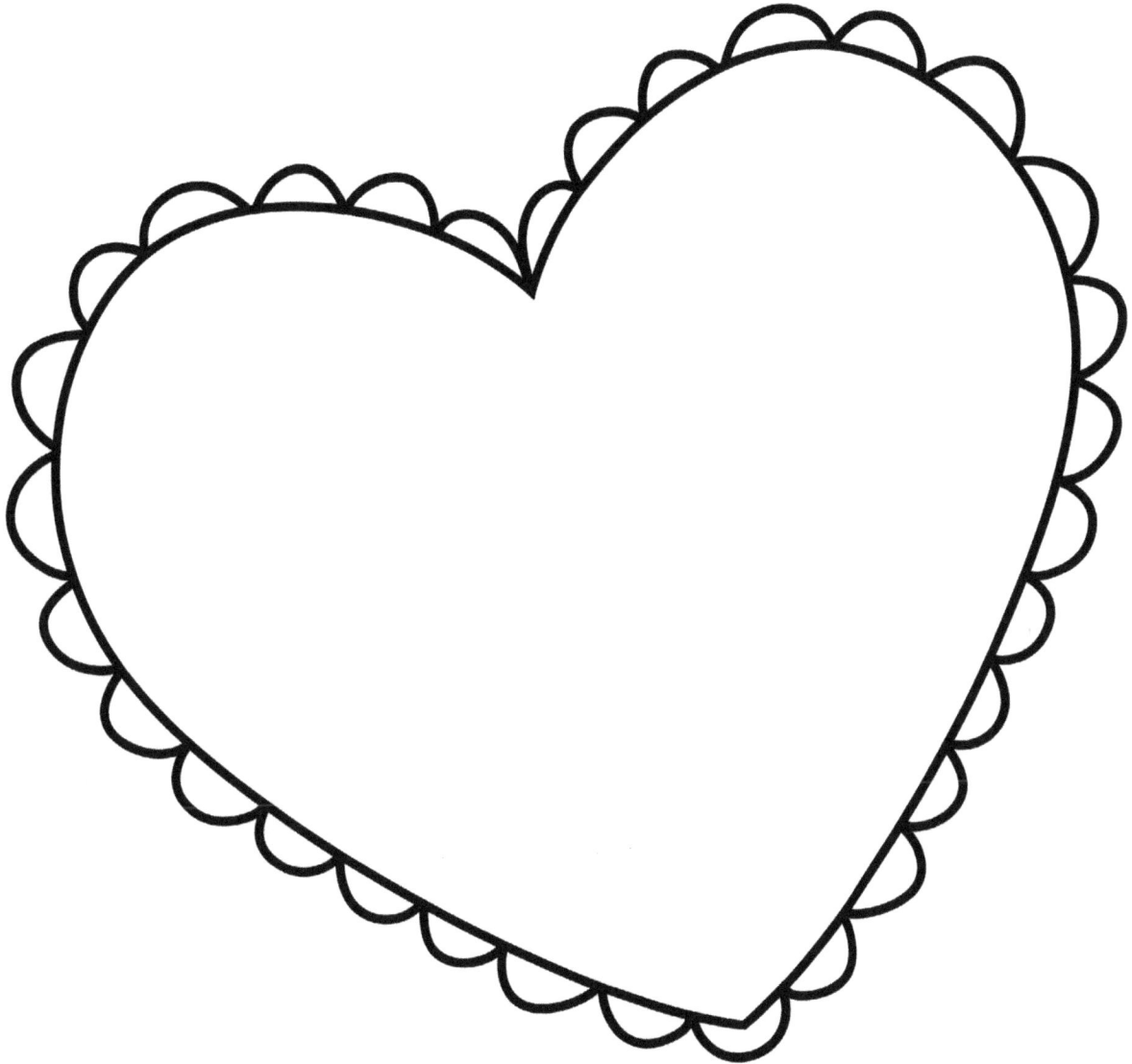

Communication

*"The more we stimulate children
and encourage communication, the
better off we are going to be."*

LINDA HURWITZ

*"Fostering communication with a child
promotes self-esteem and leads to a continuing
relationship in adolescence and into adulthood."*

NANCY KELLY

Communication is at the center of every healthy relationship. This section will discuss how to communicate about touch, consent, secrets and privacy, rejection, and establishing trust. Children will learn an assortment of ways to communicate and deal with a variety of complex issues as they learn to set boundaries and respect the boundaries of others. Many lessons in this section create an opportunity to be an askable adult for the youth in your life.

• • •

LESSON 11:
Captain May I, Consent?

Rationale:

Consent is an essential element to maintaining healthy and egalitarian relationships. This lesson will illustrate the definition of consent and cultivate the concept by putting it into practice. The importance of teaching consent to youth is so they understand consent negotiations. Being able to consent to an activity allows participants to express their own boundaries and have a clear understanding of other's boundaries and personal space. It is also important for youth to recognize how their personal emotions affect other people and how previous experiences can influence one's decision to give or deny consent.

Objectives:

- To define consent
- To illustrate and practice how to give consent

Modification for Parents/Guardians:

Trusted adults may engage in a discussion by providing specific examples of consent that are applicable to the child. Trusted adults can stress the importance of the child being able to consent to physical touch, even hugs and kisses from family members. You can also encourage your child to ask for consent, including sharing their toys with siblings or at school.

Materials:

- Chart paper

- Marker
- One sheet of green construction paper
- One sheet of red construction paper

Lesson Plan
Activity 1:

1. Explain to participants they are going to learn about something called consent. Define consent by sharing the following definition: "to give someone permission." Further explain that if they say "no" it means there is no consent.

2. Ask participants to think of times they have given other people consent. If they need an example, offer, "Think of a time your grandma, or someone else you know, asked for a hug and you gave them one, or a time when someone wanted to play with one of your toys and you agreed." List their responses on the chart paper. After listing their responses, ask, "How did it feel to give someone consent?"

3. Ask the participants to think of times they did not give consent for someone to do something, but the person did it anyway. If they need an example, offer, "Think of a time someone took a toy from you and played with it even though you told them no." Record their responses on chart paper. After listing their responses, ask, "How did it feel when you did not give someone consent?"

4. Explain to the participants that you will all play a game illustrating consent called, "Captain May I?" This classic game not only teaches participants about consent, but they also learn about boundaries and rejection. Participants will line up side by side at the opposite end of the classroom from you. If the weather allows, play the game outside. Tell participants that they will get to take turns asking if they can do something. Explain that the goal is to be the first to reach you, but they cannot move without saying, "Captain May I?," and making a request to move forward. Remind them they must also get your permission and consent and you may choose to tell them "no." Encourage participants to get creative, such as "Captain May I jump forward three times?" Continue the game play until a participant reaches you first. Congratulate the winner. If you want to play again, have the winner be the Captain. After the game, discuss the following opinion questions.

Opinion Questions for Activity 1:

- How did it feel to have to ask for consent to do something?

- How did it feel when I gave you consent?

- How did it feel when I didn't give you consent to do something?

- Why is it important to ask for consent?

Activity 2:

If time allows, you may engage in a second game called "Red Light, Green Light." Once again, ask the participants to stand up and make a line, standing side by side, at the back of the classroom. If the weather allows, play the following game outside. Once the participants have made a line, tell them you will be holding up a sign, either a red or green piece of construction paper. The red paper represents a red traffic light and the green paper represents a green traffic light. Tell them when you hold up the red paper it means STOP and the green paper means GO. Explain that if you are holding the green light, they should run towards you, but if you are holding up the red light they should stop and freeze. If the participant does not freeze at the red light, they must return to the start line. Explain this is a race, but it is also about getting consent from you to stop or go. Engage in game play. If you want to play again, have the winner be the person who holds up the red and green lights. Once again, discuss the following opinion questions.

Opinion Questions for Activity 2:

- How did it feel to have to wait for consent to stop or go?

- If you got to hold up the lights, how did it feel to have that control?

- Why is consent important?

LESSON 12:
Can I Get a Fist Bump?

Rationale:

Research from Ardiel and Rankin shows that "touch has emerged as an important modality for the facilitation of growth and development" for babies and children. Touch helps us to develop appropriate attachments, empathy, and to display emotions. A lack of touch can lead to pain, depression, and body image issues. This lesson teaches youth about the value of touch and explores when it is appropriate to touch others, how to ask for consent to touch, and how to respect the personal boundaries of others. This lesson will discuss safe and wanted touch versus unsafe and unwanted touch.

Objectives:

- To define touch as wanted or unwanted
- To explain how to ask for wanted touch
- To refuse unwanted touch
- To explain boundaries related to touch

Modification for Parents/Guardians:

This lesson is an opportunity to discuss genital touching with your child. It is common for children to touch their own genitals as a soothing technique, because it feels good or calms them down. This simple act is an association of touch and pleasure and is not sexual in nature. However, it is important to discuss boundaries with your child about genital touching and inform them it is a private act to engage in alone, usually in their bedroom or the bathtub.

Materials:

- Chart paper
- Markers

Lesson Plan:

1. Introduce the lesson by telling the participants they will be discussing touch today. Ask the group, what are the ways we touch others? What are ways we touch ourselves? Write their responses down with a marker on chart paper.

2. Ask the participants if they can share types of touch that are inappropriate, unwanted, or unsafe. Make sure to elicit responses such as hitting and kicking. Write these responses down on chart paper with a marker.

3. Next, ask the participants if they can share types of touch that feel good, safe, and wanted. Make sure to elicit responses such as hugging and giving a high five. Write all responses down on the chart paper. After they have shared all of their responses, ask if there is ever a time you don't want to be touched, even when it may be a wanted touch? If they say yes, ask them why someone might not want to be touched?

4. Tell the participants that it is important to ask for touch before we do it, to make sure it is safe and wanted. Use this opportunity to refer to Lesson #11 and ask if they remember what consent is. It is also important for other people to ask for consent or permission before touching them.

5. To practice this, ask the participants to stand up and walk around and ask their peers for a high five, a fist bump, or a hug. Tell all participants they can say yes, no, or offer one of the other options.

Opinion Questions:

- How did it feel to ask for a high five?
- How did it feel to get a high five?
- How did it feel when someone didn't want to give you a high five?
- Were there some people you felt more comfortable with? Why?

LESSON 13:
Privacy vs. Secrecy

Rationale:

Talking to kids about the differences between privacy and secrecy will help them understand boundaries. A secret may be fun for friends to share, but kids need to understand when it is a secret that a trusted adult needs to know too. Discussing privacy with kids helps them understand they can set their own boundaries about their bodies and their space, and know how to respect the boundaries of others as well. This lesson will help illustrate the differences.

Objectives:

- To define what a secret is
- To define when something is private

Modification for Parents/Guardians:

This lesson encourages you to discuss boundaries with children and discuss appropriate forms of touch. It is an opportunity to discuss genital self-touch with children. Be sure to tell them touching themselves is okay when they are alone in a private place, such as the bathroom or their bedroom. However, because it is a private activity, it should not be done in public places or shared living spaces like the car or living room. Then discuss with the child that if someone else ever asks to touch their genitals and keep this a secret, it is not okay and they should tell you right away.

Materials:

- Shoebox labeled **PRIVATE**
- Shoebox labeled **SECRET**

- Scrap paper
- Lesson 13 Handout on page 65
- Small prize or piece of candy for each participant

Lesson Plan:

1. Start the lesson by telling the participants you have something private to share. Tell them after they participate in today's lesson, you will share this information with them.

2. Tell the participants you are going to talk today about what is private and how that differs from a secret. Define a secret as information we withhold or hide from others because there may be negative consequences when shared. Define privacy as information we keep to ourselves because it is personal to us, but does not impact or hurt others.

3. Tell the participants they will be discussing six different scenarios to decide if a situation is "keeping a secret" or "keeping something private." Hand each person six pieces of scrap paper. Instruct participants to use the scrap paper to insert their vote, secret or private, into the labeled shoebox after you read each story.

4. Start by reading the first scenario (Lesson 13 Handout on page 65). When you have finished, ask the participants to cast their votes. After everyone has voted, count the pieces of paper in each shoebox to determine whether the participants voted if the story was secret or private. Then ask the participants, "How did you decide if the story was a secret or if it was private? What helped you decide?" Do this step for all six scenarios.

5. Once you have finished all six scenarios, tell the participant you are now ready to share your private information, which is that you have a prize for each of them. Then give each participant a small prize or piece of candy. After everyone has a prize, continue to the opinion questions that follow.

Opinion Questions:

- What is a secret?
- What is privacy?
- How did it feel knowing I was keeping something private the whole lesson?

- What is the difference between something private and something that's a secret?

- Is it ever okay to keep a secret?

Lesson 13 Handout

Scenario 1: Max and Ivan are playing at the playground. Max calls Ivan to the side to show him something in his pocket. He shows Ivan a rock he found. He says it is a special rock and when he rubs the rock it makes him feel calm. Max says the rock is like having superpowers. He tells Ivan not to tell anyone about his rock because he doesn't want anyone to steal it. Ivan is his best friend though, so he wanted Ivan to know about his superpowers. Is Max asking Ivan to keep the rock private or keep a secret?

Scenario 2: The entire class is outside for recess. Nakiah and Desiree are playing hopscotch by themselves. Desiree falls, skins her knees, and rips her new jeans. Nakiah says she will go get a teacher but Desiree stops her. "If the teacher sees I skinned my knees she'll call my mom and I'll get in trouble for ripping my jeans." Nakiah says Desiree didn't do anything to get in trouble but notices her knee is hurt. Desiree pleads, "My mom will think I did it for attention. Please don't tell." Is Desiree asking Nakiah to keep her fall private or keep it a secret?

Scenario 3: Cam is visiting their grandparents. Their grandfather calls them into the kitchen. He asks Cam to rub his back. He says he will give Cam a dollar if they don't tell anyone. Cam feels uncomfortable but loves their grandpa. Cam isn't sure what to do. Is Cam's grandfather asking them to keep the back rub private or keep it a secret?

Scenario 4: Jamal is out shopping with his dad. They are looking for a birthday gift for Jamal's mom. Jamal and his dad pick out the perfect gift. After they buy the gift from the store, Jamal's dad says, "Now don't tell your mother what we bought her. We want it to be a surprise when she opens it on her birthday tomorrow." Is Jamal's dad asking him to keep the gift private or keep it a secret?

Scenario 5: Alex was invited over to Gideon's for a play date. They hang out in Gideon's back yard and in the basement. Alex asks if they can go up to Gideon's room. He's sure Gideon has more toys up there to play with. Gideon says, "No, it's my space and I don't like other people to be in my room." This hurts Alex's feelings. Is Gideon keeping his bedroom private or a secret?

Scenario 6: Onyx and Madison are playing in the living room. They are having a lot of fun chasing each other and playing tag. Onyx is running a little too fast though, and knocks over a lamp. It breaks. Onyx looks at Madison and says, "Help me clean this up. Don't tell anyone I broke it though. I don't want to get in trouble." Is Onyx asking Madison to keep the breaking of the lamp private or keep it a secret?

Answer Key:

Scenario 1: Max has asked Ivan to keep this private. Max feels empowered by his rock and is not hurting himself, or anyone else, by not sharing the rock or how it makes him feel.

Scenario 2: Desiree is asking her friend to keep a secret because she tore her jeans and doesn't want to get in trouble. Nakia knows she needs to get a teacher because Desiree is hurt and her knee is bleeding.

Scenario 3: Cam's grandfather is asking him to keep a secret because Cam feels uncomfortable. In addition, Cam is being bribed with money to keep a secret.

Scenario 4: Jamal's dad has asked him to keep the gift private so it will be a surprise for his mother. Tomorrow Jamal and his father will give the mother a surprise gift.

Scenario 5: Gideon is keeping his room private. He feels protective of his personal space and is creating a boundary for himself and his toys, and his choice is not harming anyone.

Scenario 6: Onyx is asking Madison to keep a secret so they do not get in trouble for breaking the lamp. Onyx is asking Madison to lie by keeping this secret.

LESSON 14:
Reject, Reflect, Accept

Rationale:

Feeling rejected is a natural emotion, but we are not fully equipped to deal with it. While rejection can make us feel hurt, sad, or angry, it is something everyone will experience. After reflecting on feelings of rejection and working through the emotion, we may be better able to accept it. Helping youth to normalize feelings of rejection, as well as how to reject others in a healthy and respectful way, will increase emotional intelligence and awareness.

Objectives:

- To define rejection
- To illustrate handling feelings of rejection in a healthy manner
- To practice rejecting others in a delicate manner
- To illustrate not taking rejection personally

Modification for Parents/Guardians:

In addition to using the role-plays, you can discuss personal examples where your child has been rejected, or rejected others, to help cultivate displays of empathy.

Materials:

- Chart paper
- Marker
- Lesson 14 Handout on page 69

Lesson Plan:

1. Welcome the participants to today's lesson. On a piece of chart paper, draw a large circle. Within the circle, draw a bunch of small circles. Outside the large circle, draw a small circle by itself. Ask the participants what they think is happening in this drawing. What do they notice? Ask them how they think all the circles inside the large circle feel. What about the small circle by itself? Congratulate them on their observations.

2. After the circle exercise, tell the participants, "Today we will be discussing what it feels like to be left out, just like the little circle." Proceed by writing the word "Rejection" on a piece of chart paper. Ask the participants if anyone knows what the word "rejection" means. Invite all responses and write all replies on the chart paper. Explain that rejection is when someone is left out, told no, or not accepted.

3. Next, provide each participant with a handout. Tell the participants they will be engaging in a variety of role-plays to demonstrate how to handle being rejected and how to reject someone.

4. Ask for volunteers to engage in the role-plays. Give participants a few minutes to read over the role-plays and practice their acting skills. When they are ready to start acting, ask for the volunteers to begin.

5. After each role-play, discuss the following:

   ∘ How was the person in the role-play rejected?
   ∘ How did it make them feel?
   ∘ How did they handle the rejection?
   ∘ How did the person in the role-play reject someone?
   ∘ Was there anything you would have done differently if this were you?

6. Once all of the role-plays have concluded, discuss the opinion questions.

Opinion Questions:

- Can you think of a time when you were rejected? How did it make you feel? How did you handle it?

- Can you think of a time when you rejected someone? How did it make you feel? How did you handle it?

- Would you do anything different when being rejected or when rejecting someone after today's lesson? What would you do differently? How? Why? (You may choose to record their responses on chart paper.)

Lesson 14 Handout

Role Playing

1. Christian and Aden are good friends at school and enjoy playing together on the playground during recess. Today, Aden was invited to play soccer on the field with some other kids. Christian was not. Aden really wants to play soccer with new friends today. How is Aden feeling? What can Aden say to Christian? How will Christian react?

2. Dylan and Robert are in the same grade. They have a lot of fun at school and have arranged a sleepover at Dylan's house. Dylan's brother Terrell is a year younger than they are. Terrell and Dylan get along well and like to play the same games together. Dylan and Robert have already started a game and are laughing. Terrell sees them having fun and wants to play too. What can Terrell say to them? What will Dylan and Robert say to Terrell? Do you think they should include Terrell in the sleepover? Why or why not?

3. Ebony and Ericka like to sit at the same lunch table and share snacks. Ebony doesn't want to sit with Ericka today because she is upset with her. Ebony blames Ericka for missing morning recess because they were whispering to one another and got caught by their teacher. What should Ebony tell Ericka about lunch today? How will Ericka react?

4. Stella and Wilson have been friends since kindergarten. Stella is having a birthday party next week but didn't invite Wilson because her friends told her, "Boys have cooties." Wilson just found out he wasn't invited to the party. How is Wilson feeling? What will he say to Stella? What will Stella do?

5. Isaiah and Juliette are both running for class president. Juliette wins and is very excited. Isaiah is very sad to have lost and feels like their classmates do not like them. What can Juliette say to Isaiah? Is there something their teacher could say? What about Isaiah's other classmates? Should Isaiah say anything to anyone about how they are feeling? Who should Isaiah talk to?

6. Miracle has four siblings. She loves to run errands with her mother so she can spend time alone with her. Today, Miracle's mother asked Miracle's little brother Antonio to run errands, and Miracle has to stay home and babysit her other siblings. How do you think Miracle is feeling? What will she do? What can she say to her mother? What could her mother say to make her feel better?

LESSON 15:
Trusting Me, Trusting You

Rationale:

Establishing a sense of trust is essential to a child's upbringing and growth. Trusting others, and oneself, helps children develop a positive self-image, friendships, and confidence. It also helps create secure attachments in relationships. This exercise is a lesson in trust that is both fun and engaging for youth.

Objectives:

- To define what trust is
- To illustrate trusting others and yourself

Modification for Parents/Guardians:

This lesson helps instill a sense of trust in your child. To modify this lesson, you may choose to have your child wear the blindfold and do this exercise to trust you, and then reverse roles so you can illustrate that you also trust your child. Use this as a time to talk to your child about the importance of trusting you and why it is equally important you trust them.

Materials:

- Chart paper
- Marker
- Blindfold
- Gold coins or another small toy

Lesson Plan:

1. Begin the lesson by welcoming the participants and saying, "Do you trust me? Why or why not?" or "Think about someone you trust. Now think about someone you don't trust. Why do you trust or not trust them?" You may get a variety of responses. Acknowledge their reasons for trusting you, or not. Thank the participants for their responses.

2. Label a piece of chart paper, "Trust." Ask the participants, "What are the things you need to trust someone?" Record their responses on the chart paper. Ask, "What are the things you do to earn trust?" Add those responses to the chart paper.

3. Tell the participants they are going to play a game that is based on trust. You will need one volunteer from the group to help complete a treasure hunt. This volunteer will need to wear the blindfold.

4. The rest of the participants should each get a gold coin or small toy. The coins are the treasure. Have them hide the coins throughout the room while the volunteer is wearing the blindfold. Once they have all been hidden, tell the volunteer they are going on a treasure hunt but they will have to trust their peers to help them find the gold. Tell the participants they need to trust that the volunteer will find the hidden gold coins.

5. The participants will help their peers find the treasure by giving them clues, telling them when they are close to the gold, if they need to bend down or reach higher to find it, etc. Have the participants take turns to help their peers find five to seven gold coins. There will be a lot more coins scattered so the volunteer has a high chance of finding a few. If there is time, have another volunteer put on the blindfold and trust their peers to find the treasure.

6. Once they have finished playing the game, because they have found all of the gold coins or are out of time, move on to the opinion questions and congratulate the group on trusting one another.

Opinion Questions:

- Ask the volunteers, what was it like trusting your peers to find the gold coins? What made it easy? What made it difficult?

- Ask the rest of the participants, did you trust your peer would find the gold coins? What made you trust they would find the coins? What made you think they might not find the coins?
- Who do you trust the most?
- Do you trust yourself?

Diversity

*"It is time for parents to teach young people early
on that in diversity there is beauty and strength."*

MAYA ANGELOU

Inspired by Angelou's quote, this section dives into diversity and explores same-sex relationships, privilege, religion, transgender youth, and abilities. Children are given the opportunity to learn about how people may be different, and how to embrace and honor them instead of othering them. At the heart of each diversity lesson is a message on inclusion. With a focus on inclusion, we strive towards equity and dismantling oppressive systems among the varying identities within sexuality.

• • •

LESSON 16:
My Mom's a Cat

Rationale:

This lesson[1] will utilize the book *And Tango Makes Three* by Justin Richardson and Peter Parnell. Participants will read the book, which illustrates a real-life example of same-sex parenting. The participants will discuss their own families as a means of recognizing various household infrastructures. After reading the book and engaging in a discussion, participants will write down the names of their family members and assign an animal that describes each member. This activity will illustrate that everyone's family looks different, as well as create a personal connection to the book.

Objectives:

- Identify components of a family
- Define same-sex parents
- Describe how their own family dynamics are unique from other people
- Identify how their personal life relates to the story in the book

Modification for Parents/Guardians:

Encourage a discussion with your child about your own family dynamics.

Materials:

- Book or video reading of *And Tango Makes Three*
- Markers, crayons, or colored pencils
- Lesson 16 Handout on page 81

....

1 This lesson was adapted from *My Mom's a Cat* by Kristen Lilla and Christian Hoeger, published by The Center for Sex Education manual *Orientation: Teaching about Identity, Attraction, & Behavior,* Volume 2, 2020, pages 167–170.

Lesson Plan:

1. Have the group sit in a position where everyone can see the book from where you will be standing or sitting.

2. Explain that the group is going to read a book today called *And Tango Makes Three*. Explain that today's lesson will focus on how everyone's family is different.

3. Read the book aloud to the group. Be sure to show the group pictures from the book.

4. After reading the book, discuss the following opinion questions:

   ◦ Who were Tango's parents in this story?
   ◦ How do you know they were Tango's parents?
   ◦ Who else was part of Tango's family?
   ◦ Who makes a family?
   ◦ Who helps raise you?

5. As needed based on their answers, explain to participants that, just like Tango's family, everyone's family is different. Elaborate that some participants may be raised by a single parent, some are raised by their grandparents, and some may be raised by two moms or two dads, just like Tango.

6. Provide participants with an explanation that Tango's parents are the same gender and introduce the word *gay*. Provide this definition of gay: being sexually attracted to someone who is the same gender.

7. Have participants move to desks or tables. Provide each participant with a handout and coloring utensils. A participant may need more than one handout if they have a large family.

8. Have participants read the directions at the top of the handout. Ask for any questions, then have them complete the handout. Encourage their personal creativity and ideas.

9. Invite participants to share their drawings with the group and explain why they assigned particular animals to each person. Ask why each person in their family is not the same animal.

10. Ask participants the following questions, while emphasizing that all families are made up of different kinds of people, with different personalities, genders, and dynamics.

Opinion Questions:

- What makes your family different from other people's families?

- How is your family like Tango's?

- What might you say to someone with a family that is different from yours?

Lesson 16 Handout

Directions: Write the names of your family members on the lines in the boxes. Now draw a picture of an animal in the box that reminds you of that family member.

Me

_____

_____

_____

_____

LESSON 17:
Colors of You

Rationale:

This lesson will define race and ethnicity so students can learn new definitions. They will learn about melanin, and how this is the driving factor in determining skin color. Students will also learn the acronym BIPOC (Black and Indigenous People of Color). Once they have an understanding of these words, students will do an art project to create images of themselves to help illustrate how skin tone varies from person to person. Students will have the opportunity to discuss how they see race in the world, including how they have seen people treated differently based on the color of their skin. The lesson will conclude by teaching participants how to begin being anti-racist.

Objectives:

- Define race and ethnicity
- Define melanin
- Define BIPOC
- Define racism
- Discuss observations about skin tone and how to be anti-racist

Modification for Parents/Guardians:

This lesson is an opportunity for you to discuss race and ethnicity with your child. Help your child understand their race, and identify other people in the world who look similar to them. (Perhaps this includes you.) Discuss with your child whether they have ever been treated differently for any reason. Hold space for this conversation, even if it is difficult, as it creates a safe space for your child to discuss experiencing or witnessing racism. If your child is white, encourage a discussion about privilege and how their skin tone affords them this and how they can be anti-racist. *Race Cars* by Jenny Devenny is a great book about race and white privilege that helps explain this difficult concept to children.

Materials:

- Chart paper
- Yarn in a variety of colors, including brown, black, yellow, and orange
- Glue
- Paper plates
- Markers
- Crayons or paint in a variety of shades, including brown, yellow, white, and black
- Optional:
  - Paintbrushes
  - Google eyes
  - Book: *If You Lived When There Was Slavery in America*

Lesson Plan:

1. Welcome the class and write the words race, ethnicity, melanin, and BIPOC on different pieces of chart paper. Ask the class if anyone can define these words. Welcome all answers and acknowledge these can be difficult words to define.

2. Define each word for the class. According to Tiffany Jewell, "When we talk about race, we are referring to our skin color" while "ethnicity zeroes in on your family's cultural and ancestral heritage." Explain that melanin is a chemical found in the body. People with more melanin have darker skin, and people with less melanin have lighter skin and freckles. Explain the final word, BIPOC, is actually an acronym for "Black and Indigenous People of Color." Share that when someone says they are BIPOC, they are describing their race.

3. Explain that each student will now create an art project where they will create a picture of a person. They may choose to create a picture of themselves or get creative and have fun making art. Provide each student with a paper plate and have them draw a face on it. Use the paint and brushes to

paint "skin," or have them use crayons to color on the plate. Next, have each student select a hair color and cut yarn. Encourage them to twist, braid, or tie the yarn to create a hairstyle they like and glue it on the plate. Finally, if you opted for google eyes, have the students glue them on the plate.

4. Have the students showcase their art projects. You may choose to have them line their plates from lightest to darkest, to show how much skin tone varies, since no two pictures will be the same.

5. Tell the class that race is a significant part of a person's identity because it is something we can see on the outside. Explain that some people are treated differently, and poorly, because they have darker skin. This is called "racism." Elaborate: "Our goal is for everyone to be anti-racist so people will be treated fairly. Tiffany Jewell says, "An anti-racist person is someone who is opposed to racism. Anti-racism is actively working against racism. It is making a commitment to resisting unjust laws, policies, and racist attitudes.""

6. Ask the students if they have ever seen racism, or experienced racism. Before you invite any responses, explain that white people do not experience racism. You can validate that everyone, regardless of skin tone, may have experienced stereotypes and poor treatment, but white people have advantages others do not and cannot experience racism. If you need an example, you can share that it was primarily BIPOC people who were enslaved, and that white people owned slaves. You may choose to read *If You Lived When There Was Slavery in America* by Anne Kamma to discuss this history further.

7. Write "anti-racism" on a piece of chart paper. Define anti-racism once again to the class. Ask participants to list ways they can be anti-racist. Invite all ideas and be sure to implement them in your classroom so you are also role-modeling anti-racism. Once you are done brainstorming anti-racist ideas, discuss the opinion questions.

Opinion Questions:

- What is the difference between race and ethnicity?
- What does it mean to be anti-racist?
- What is an example of being anti-racist?

LESSON 18:
A World of Religion

Rationale:

There are thousands of religions around the world. We have come to refer to the largest and most well-known religions as the "Big Five." These include Christianity, Judaism, Islam, Buddhism, and Hinduism. This lesson teaches youth about different religions and encourages acceptance of other faith systems.

Objectives:

- To explain the Big Five
- To identify the main beliefs of each of the Big Five
- To explain a holiday meal from each of the Big Five

Modification for Parents/Guardians:

This lesson is an opportunity to explain your own beliefs and values to your child regarding your faith, religion, or spiritual beliefs. It is also a chance to help children understand other people's religious faith and belief systems. You may want to revisit this lesson on the religious holidays discussed. When the holiday occurs, you can talk about the faith again and make one of the meals suggested to learn more about the culture.

Materials:

- Chart paper
- Markers
- Lesson 18 Handout on page 89

Lesson Plan:

1. Welcome the group and tell them they will be learning about religion today. Tell them there are five main world religions, known as the "Big Five." Ask the participants, "Can you name the Big Five?" Write their responses down on chart paper with a marker. If they do not think of all five religions, help the participants and write them on the chart paper. The Big Five include: Christianity, Judaism, Islam, Buddhism, and Hinduism. Ask the students to share if they or their family practice any religion or beliefs not listed as part of the Big Five.

2. Tell the participants they will be learning more about each religion and you will share some facts with them. Provide each participant with The Big Five handout which explains the main points and holiday(s) of each religion.

3. Make a dish from one of the following suggestions. Please note recipes may vary by region and location in the world.

   ◦ **Christianity:** ham, deviled eggs, gingerbread cookies, eggnog
   ◦ **Islam:** bolani, samosas
   ◦ **Hinduism:** kheer, gulab jamun
   ◦ **Buddhism:** steamed kuih, fried meehoon
   ◦ **Judaism:** apples and honey, challah bread, matzo ball soup, gefilte fish

4. If unable to make or provide food, modify this lesson by having the class make decorations from each of the Big Five's major holidays. Split the class into five groups, having each group work on a different decoration and then present it to the class.

5. When you have finished discussing The Big Five and activity, have participants discuss the following opinion questions.

Opinion Questions:

- What is something you learned today about religion?
- What similarities did you notice about The Big Five?
- What differences did you notice about The Big Five?
- How does your family celebrate holidays?
- What special foods do you eat on holidays?

Lesson 18 Handout

The Big Five

Christianity is the world's largest religion. Christians believe that a man named Jesus is the Son of God. The religion is over 2,000 years old. Christians learn religious text from the Bible. The main holidays Christians celebrate include Easter (when Jesus rose from the dead) and Christmas (Jesus' birthday). On Easter, it is common to eat ham and deviled eggs. On Christmas in the United States, it is common to eat gingerbread cookies and drink eggnog.

Islam is the world's second largest religion. It is over 1,500 years old. People of Islam faith believe in one God and believe a man named Muhammad served as God's messenger. Followers of Islam learn religious text from the Quran. In Islam, the main holidays are Ramadan (to honor when Muhammad delivered text for the Quran) and Eid-Al Adha (Festival of the Sacrifice). During Ramadan people fast, or do not eat during the day. When the sun goes down it is common to break the fast by eating samosas (fried stuffed dough) or Bolani (stuffed flat bread).

Hinduism is the third largest religion in the world. It is about 2,500 years old. The Hindus learn religious text from Vedas. Hinduism is most common in India and parts of Asia. The Hindus believe in truth. They also believe in many gods and goddesses. In fact, they believe in 33 million gods. The main holidays in Hinduism are Diwali (Festival of Lights) and Dussehra (celebrating good over evil). During Diwali it is common to eat sweets such as kheer and gulab jamun. People might eat kheer during Dussehra too.

Buddhism is the fourth largest religion in the world. It is 6,000–8,000 years old. Buddhist people believe in the cycle of death and rebirth. Buddhists learn religious texts from Sanskrit. The Buddhists do not believe in a God. They follow the path of Buddha, who was a monk and teacher. The main holidays in Buddhism are Vesak (celebrating the life of Buddha) and Parinirvana Day (the day Buddha died). On Vesak, Buddhists do not eat meat, but it is common to eat steamed kuih (cake) or fried meehoon (noodles).

Judaism is over 4,000 years old and the fifth largest religion in the world. At the time, many people worshiped numerous gods. Jewish people believe in only one God. They believe that a man named Abraham encouraged the Jewish faith.

Jewish people learn religious text from the Torah. The main holidays are Rosh Hashanah (the Jewish New Year), Yom Kippur (Day of Atonement where people ask for forgiveness for any wrongdoing they have done), and Passover, or Pesach (celebration of freedom from slavery). On Rosh Hashanah people eat apples and honey. For Yom Kippur people fast all day and do not eat. When they break the fast, they may eat challah bread. On Passover it is common to eat gefilte fish and matzo ball soup.

LESSON 19:
Transgender and Non-Binary Youth

Rationale:

Research collected from the Williams Institute estimates there are 1.6 million people ages 13 and up who identify as transgender. Many youths reject the limitations of the binary of being a girl or a boy. Youth have felt safer coming out as transgender and non-binary in recent years. Despite more acceptance and education, transgender youth still have higher rates of depression, suicide, and substance abuse than their heterosexual counterparts. It is imperative to help reduce these rates, be an active ally, and show acceptance for youth struggling with their gender journey.

Objectives:

- To define the term transgender
- To define the term non-binary
- To illustrate what it means to be a transgender or non-binary youth

Modification for Parents/Guardians:

You may choose to do this lesson with your child on Trans Day of Visibility on March 31 or during Pride month in June. You could take your child to a local event, such as a Pride parade, so they can see you being an active ally. If you or your child is transgender, this is an opportunity to discuss together. This is also an opportunity to explain the history of Pride, which started in 1970 after the Stonewall Riots.

Materials:

- Book or video reading of *I Am Jazz* by Jazz Jennings
- Optional reading: *A Princess of Great Daring* by S. Bear Bergman
- Lesson 19 Handout on page 95
- Crayons or colored pencils

Lesson Plan:

1. Introduce the lesson today by telling participants they will be learning about a special kid named Jazz. Tell the participants they will be learning more about Jazz and her life.

2. Introduce the book *I am Jazz,* or find a video reading online. Ask participants to listen and look at the pictures, and save their questions until the end. Read, or listen to the book.

3. Once you have finished the book, be sure to define the term transgender for the participants. Explain that someone who is transgender may be born with a vulva and feel like a boy or be born with a penis and feel like a girl, just like Jazz. This may be an opportunity to connect lessons #1–5 within this lesson. Continue explaining that some kids don't really feel like a boy or a girl, or they may feel like both, and they identify as non-binary. Explain that being transgender or non-binary is not the same as engaging in activities that do not fit a gender stereotype.

4. Allow the children to ask questions and share feedback about the book and the new definitions you offered. Answer any questions you can. If you don't know the answer to a question they have, be honest and say, "I don't know."

5. Tell the participants that Jazz is proud of who she is and has pride. Explain that other kids like Jazz celebrate pride all year long, but the month of June is dedicated to celebrating Pride each year. Elaborate that Pride is about being proud of who you are! (If time allows, you may choose to share the history of Pride, which started in 1970 after the Stonewall Riots.)

6. Provide each participant with a handout of a blank flag. Tell them the colors of the Pride flag are the colors of the rainbow, and the colors of the Transgender flag are pink, blue, and white. Now tell them to each create their own Pride flag using crayons or colored pencils.

7. Once all of the participants have finished coloring their own Pride flags, ask them to share with the group and explain what their flag means. When everyone has had a chance to share, move on to the opinion questions.

Opinion Questions:

- Can someone tell me what the word transgender means?
- Can someone tell me what the word non-binary means?
- How do you think it felt for Jazz to find out about the word transgender?
- What makes Jazz special?
- What makes you feel proud and prideful?

Lesson 19 Handout

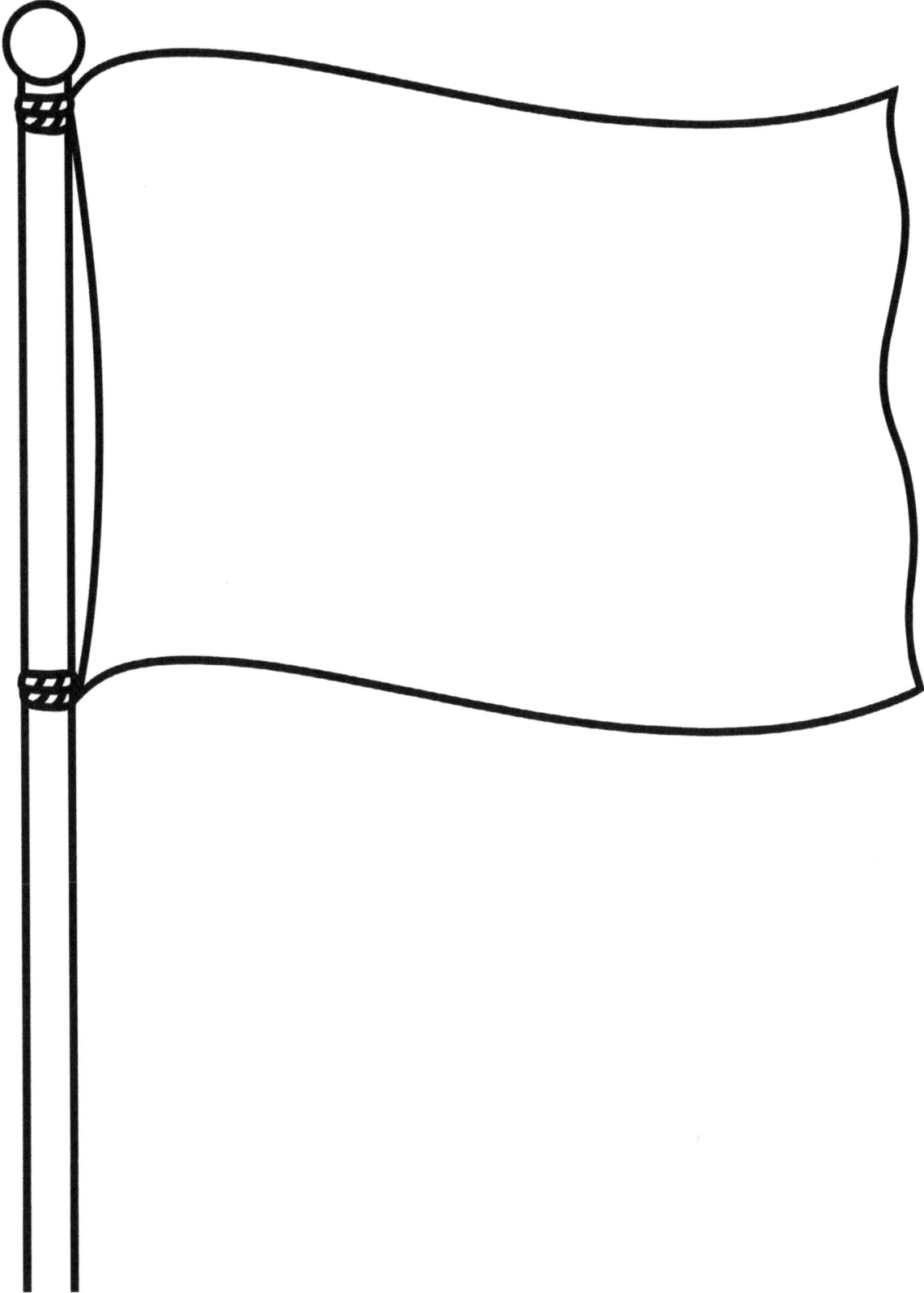

LESSON 20:
The Five Senses

Rationale:

People have five senses: sight, touch, hearing, taste, and smell. When one of these senses, or abilities, is affected, a person has a disability. Disabilities affect millions of people in the world. Teaching youth to appreciate their own abilities and to accept the abilities of others will allow them to interact in a patient and non-judgmental way. It creates a space for participants to interact differently with their peers who have disabilities and find ways to be more inclusive. It is also important to note that not all disabilities can be seen, and it is important to help children understand the concept of invisible disabilities too (such as autism or dyslexia). This activity also helps foster youth's sensory development.

Objectives:

- To define the five senses
- To understand what each of the senses does

Modification for Parents/Guardians:

If you are the trusted adult of a child with disabilities, you may modify this lesson to help them understand why peers may be curious about their disability. Encourage them to find ways to discuss their disability, or to find ways to set boundaries regarding this conversation as they are entitled to not share their experiences. If you have a child with no disabilities, help instill a lesson of acceptance and patience. Discuss real-life examples of people you may know who have a disability, to help personalize this lesson for your child. Be sure to do the activity and then discuss it with them too!

Materials:

- Chart paper
- Marker
- Headphones
- Tablet/computer/phone
- Three jars wrapped in foil
- Three boxes
- Blindfold
- Magnifying glass

Please note *all* items may be modified for this exercise. The following are just suggestions.

- Items for hearing
  - Sound of crickets chirping
  - Sound of water dripping
  - Sound of wood floor creaking
- Items for sight
  - Flowers
  - Leaves
  - Small piece of wood with grain
- Items for smell
  - Coffee beans
  - Vinegar
  - Flowers
- Items for touch
  - Silky fabric
  - Bowl of cooked noodles
  - Rock
- Items for taste
  - Salty (a pretzel, for example)
  - Sweet (candy, for example)
  - Sour (lemon, for example)
  - Optional: water

Lesson Plan:

1. Introduce the lesson to the participants by telling them they will be learning about their different abilities today. Ask the participants, what is an ability? Accept all answers offered.

2. Next, ask the participants if they have heard of the five senses. Share with them that all five senses are abilities we have. Note that sometimes people have a *dis*ability and not all five of their senses work the same way. Tell the participants that in order to learn more about their own abilities they will be learning about all of the senses today.

3. Ask the participants if they can name all five senses. Write their responses down on chart paper with a marker. If any of their responses include one of the five senses, circle it. Share any missed senses with participants, write them on the chart paper, and circle them. You should now have all five senses listed: **hearing, sight, smell, touch, taste.**

4. For the hands-on exercise, you may choose to split the participants into five small groups or keep them as one group. If you have a large group, it is recommended you split the participants up. Have five stations set up around the room, one for each activity.

5. At the **hearing** station you should have headphones and a tablet/computer/phone setup. Participants should put on the headphones and listen to the sounds of crickets chirping, then water dripping, and finally a wood floor creaking. Ask the participants if they can identify the sounds they are listening to.

6. At the **sight** station there should be a magnifying glass and flowers. Have the participants look at the flowers, leaves, and a small piece of wood with grain. What do they notice about them? Then have the participants use the magnifying glass to look closer at each item. What details do they notice now?

7. At the **smell** station, you should have three foil-wrapped jars filled with strongly scented things such as coffee beans, vinegar, and flowers. The foil is wrapped around the jar so participants cannot see what they are about to smell. Take the lid off of the jars and have the participants inhale deeply. What do they smell? Do they like the smell? Dislike it? What does it remind them of?

8. At the **touch** station, you should have three boxes. Each box should be filled with items such as silk fabric, cooked noodles, and a rock. Have the participants put their hand into the box and touch the item. What do they feel? Can they identify what it is?

9. At the **taste** station, participants should put on a blindfold so they cannot see what food items are in front of them. You should have something salty, something sweet, and something bitter for participants to taste. You may want to have water at this station so participants can cleanse their palate after each food item. Have participants take a bite of each food item, one at a time. Can they identify what they are eating? Can they describe the taste? Encourage them to use words like salty, sweet, and sour.

10. After participants have gone to each table, have them come back together as a group and answer the opinion questions together.

Opinion Questions:

- What did you learn from going to all of the stations?
- Have you ever had an experience where one of your five senses didn't work as well?
- How do you think your senses all work together?
- What are some invisible disabilities?
- How might we treat someone who has a disability or different abilities than our own?

Emotions

"The best and most beautiful things in the world cannot be seen or even touched. They must be felt with the heart."

HELEN KELLER

Identifying and expressing emotions are skills that must be taught and practiced like any other skill. This can be difficult for children as they try to understand how they are feeling, how to express those feelings, and subsequently how to manage a range of emotions. This section includes a variety of lessons to help children identify and articulate their own feelings and to honor the feelings of others. Children will have an opportunity to learn how to express emotions verbally and through body language. It is through learning these important skills about emotions and feelings that help one develop a greater sense of identity.

• • •

LESSON 21:
Climbing the Emotional Ladder

Rationale:

We all experience a wide range of emotions. Kids often have a more difficult time regulating their emotions, so they often seem dramatic, such as having a tantrum when they are frustrated or angry, and being hyper when they are excited. Helping kids recognize there is a range of emotions for each feeling, from big to small and everything in between, will help them regulate their own emotional state.

Objectives:

- To illustrate a range of emotions
- To identify coping skills and how to regulate emotions

Modification for Parents/Guardians:

To reinforce this lesson, parents can check in about their child's emotions. For example, ask the child which number their emotion is between one and three. This can be particularly useful when a child is having a big emotion, at a three, because it will force them to stop and think, thus regulating the emotion.

Materials:

- Painter tape
- Chart paper
- Marker

Lesson Plan:

1. Before the lesson begins, use the painter tape to make a "ladder" with four "steps." The first line is the bottom of the ladder or calming space, the second line is Little, the third line is Medium, and the last line is Big.

2. Welcome the participants by sharing an emotion you are feeling. You might say, "I am happy to see you all today." Tell them they will be talking about emotions today. Ask them to list any emotions they can think of. List them on the chart paper labeled "Emotions/Feelings."

3. Next, introduce the five emotions they will be talking about today: happy, sad, angry, fear, and jealousy. Circle them on the chart paper if they were listed. Write any they missed on the chart paper.

4. Tell the participants they will be playing a game to learn more about these five emotions and how they are expressed. Have them all stand at the bottom of the "ladder" and take a deep breath in through the nose and out through the mouth. (You can also have them place their hands on their hearts.) To explain the game, do an example as a group. Ask the participants, "What makes you a little bit sad?" Elicit a few responses. Have them all step to the first line of tape, then ask them what being a little bit sad looks like. As they begin to make a sad face, explain this is what a little emotion looks like. Have everyone go back to the bottom of the ladder and ask everyone to take a deep breath in and slowly let it out, reminding the group we can always use our breath to "come back down the ladder." Next you can ask, "What makes you medium sad?" Elicit a few responses. Have everyone step to the second line of tape and ask them to show you what it looks like to feel medium sad. After they show you, have participants go back to the beginning of the ladder. Again, have everyone take a deep breath in and slowly let it out. The last question, is "What does it look like when someone is very sad and has a big emotion?" Once they walk to the final ladder step and display this, again have them go back to the beginning to take as many deep breaths as they need to "come back down the ladder" and regulate their emotions.

5. Use the ladder and steps to go through each emotion: happy, sad, anger, fear, jealousy. If you have a large group, you may choose to have five participants do one emotion at a time and have the rest sit and observe. For example, in a group of 25, each group can do one emotion. Be sure to have them take a

deep breath in and out after expressing each emotion. For the big emotions, it is likely the kids will be dramatic and silly.

6. Once the participants have gone through all five emotions of happiness, sadness, anger, fear, and jealousy, have them sit in a circle or back at their desks and discuss the opinion questions.

Opinion Questions:

- Why did we take a deep breath after expressing each emotion?
- What differences did you notice about little, medium, and big emotions?
- Did you notice that when people have a big emotion, they all look similar? How so? Why do you think that is?
- What helps you bring a big emotion down to a little one?
- What do you do when you see someone else having a big emotion?

LESSON 22:
Feelings Charades

Rationale:

Communication occurs in many ways, including verbally (verbal), through physical touch (nonverbal), body language (visual), or with pen and paper (written). With so many different ways to communicate our emotions, we may not always make it clear to others what we are feeling. Expressing emotions can be difficult. Understanding what others are feeling can be even more difficult. Learning to understand facial expressions and body language can help create compassion, empathy and healthier relationships.

Objectives:

- To illustrate different emotions
- To describe non-verbal body language and facial expressions

Modification for Parents/Guardians:

You could make this lesson part of family game night. After the game, encourage your kids to talk about their feelings with you.

Materials:

- Lesson 22 Handout on page 109

Lesson Plan:

1. Welcome the participants using a feeling. For example, "I am so happy to have you all here today. I am feeling excited about our lesson." Ask the participants how they are feeling today. Welcome all responses.

2. Tell the participants they will be discussing feelings today. Ask if anyone can define what a feeling is. It is likely someone will respond "an emotion." If they do not, share this synonym.

3. Tell the participants they are going to learn more about emotions and feelings today by playing a game of Feelings Charades. Make sure you have cut each of the Feelings from the handout separately and put them in a container. Explain the rules of the game to the participants.

   ○ Select a volunteer. This person will take a feeling out of the container.
   ○ The volunteer will read the feeling on the paper to themself but will not tell anyone else what it says.
   ○ Using acting skills, act out the feeling, but do not talk to give clues.
   ○ The rest of the participants will guess what feeling is being acted out.
   ○ The person who guesses correctly will get to act out the next feeling.

4. When you have completed all of the feelings cards, discuss the opinion questions as a group.

Opinion Questions:

- What was difficult about guessing someone else's feelings?
- What was easy about guessing someone else's feelings?
- Would it have been easier if the person acting could talk? Why?
- Why is it important to talk about how we are feeling?
- What could you do if you weren't sure how someone else was feeling?

Lesson 22 Handout

Take the time to cut out each square individually.

HAPPY	SAD	ANGRY
PROUD	SCARED	CONFIDENT
LONELY	GUILTY	SILLY
SURPRISED	JEALOUS	WORRIED
NERVOUS	SHY	CONFUSED

LESSON 23:
I Feel...

Rationale:

Identifying how we are feeling is the first step to being able to regulate our emotional state. Once emotions are identified and regulated, we can then choose how to express them appropriately. The ways in which we identify and express our feelings is a key communication skill that helps us develop good relationships.

Objectives:

- To illustrate how to express emotions
- To identify how one is feeling given their emotional state

Modification for Parents/Guardians:

Encourage children to articulate their emotional state on a consistent basis. This will help them stop and engage in mindfulness as they learn to identify and express their emotions. You can also use this as a validating experience for your child so they know expressing a range of emotions is healthy and okay. Take it a step further and share with your child how you are feeling. You may even consider doing a daily check-in, asking, "What feelings did you experience today?" Acknowledge that we experience a range of emotions on any given day. If your child is struggling to identify their emotions, get a feelings poster and help them match their feelings with the facial expressions shown on the poster.

Materials:

- Lesson 23 Handout on page 113
- Optional book: *My Body Sends a Signal* by Natalia Maguire

Lesson Plan:

1. To start today's lesson, welcome the participants and ask everyone to stand if they can. Ask everyone to show you how they are feeling today, without using their words. See if you can guess how a few people are feeling.

2. Next, ask the entire group to act out being happy, without using words or sounds. After this, have them act out being sad without using their words. Finally, have them express anger without using words. Have participants take a seat and tell them they did a great job acting out emotions.

3. While expressing emotions with facial expressions and body language is important, it is just as important to use our words. Tell the participants they will be practicing additional ways to express their emotions today, and also practice learning how to ask others how they are feeling and how to support them. At this point in the lesson, you may choose to read the optional book, *My Body Sends a Signal* by Natalia Maguire, about identifying and expressing emotions.

4. This lesson includes six role-plays to act out. Explain to the participants that role-play is acting, just like how they acted out their emotions when the lesson began today. You will need a total of 12 volunteers, two for each role-play. If you would like to have everyone participate, you can do a role-play more than once with different actors. Each time a role-play is done, it will be performed differently and will give the participants more to talk about.

5. Choose your volunteers. You can give them the role-play or you can read the role-play to the volunteers. Inform volunteers that their job as actors is to express and communicate feelings and listen to how others are feeling. The feeling described in each role-play is italicized. Go through all six role-plays, discussing the opinion questions after each one.

Opinion Questions:

- What was it like to act out different feelings? Was it easy? Hard?

- What helped you find out how someone else was feeling in the role-play?

- Is it easy or hard to share your feelings with others in real life? What makes it easier? When is it more difficult?

- Do you tend to use your words to express how you are feeling, or do you prefer facial expressions and body language? Which do you think is more effective in communicating how you feel?

Lesson 23 Handout

Role Playing

Scenario 1: Taylor just received good news and is very *happy*. This morning her mother told her she is going on a summer vacation to an amusement park and gets to bring a friend. Isha comes over to play and can tell that Taylor is *excited* about something. How will she find out what Taylor is *happy* about? Will Isha be *happy* too? What other emotions might Isha have?

Scenario 2: Liz arrives at school and sees Shawna in the corner with her head down, crying and looking *sad*. Shawna forgot her lunch that day. Liz wants to find out if Shawna is okay, so she walks over to the corner to talk to her. How will Liz find out how Shawna is feeling? How will Liz feel after talking to Shawna? How will Shawna feel about sharing?

Scenario 3: Marcus comes home from school and sees his little sister Aries sitting on the couch. She looks *angry*. Marcus is worried she is *angry* with him because he didn't walk home with her after school today. How can Marcus find out how Aries is feeling? If she is *angry* with him, how will she react when he approaches her? If she is *angry* about something else, will she talk to Marcus about it? What can Marcus do?

Scenario 4: David is having a sleepover with Nathan. When it is time to go to bed, Nathan says he is going to shut the lights off. David is *scared* of the dark. How can he explain this to Nathan before the lights are turned off? Will Nathan understand?

Scenario 5: Eric comes to school with a new blue ball. Jayleen sees Eric showing it to the other kids. Last week, Jayleen told Eric she wanted a blue ball, and now Eric has the ball she wants. Jayleen is feeling *jealous* of Eric's new ball. Should Jayleen tell him? Did Eric try to make her *jealous* on purpose?

Scenario 6: Ruby and Mara have to give a presentation for the school science fair. Mara is feeling excited to share their science project but Ruby is feeling *nervous*. Mara can tell that Ruby is *upset* about something but isn't sure what. How will Mara find out how Ruby is feeling? How can Mara support her *nervous* friend and help calm her nerves down?

114 · COLORS of YOU

LESSON 24:
Mindfulness Magic

Rationale:

Mindfulness is about being present in the moment, or finding a way to bring ourselves back to the present moment. It takes practice and patience, but mindfulness can be used as a grounding technique when a person feels overwhelmed, anxious, scared, sad, or angry. Mindfulness can be particularly useful for children to assist them in developing coping skills and to regulate their emotions.

Objectives:

- Define mindfulness
- Illustrate being in a state of mindfulness

Modification for Parents/Guardians:

You can continue practicing mindfulness with your child by making it part of your daily or weekly routine. There are many books, apps, and videos available for guided mindfulness practices. Suggested books include *My Magic Breath* by Nick Ortner, *Listening to My Body* by Gabi Garcia, and *I Can Handle It* by Laurie Wright.

Materials:

- Crayons or markers
- White paper
- Optional: Lesson 24 Handout on page 119
- Optional: Background music

Lesson Plan:

1. Welcome the participants by telling them they will be practicing something called mindfulness which encourages them to slow down, pay attention to their surroundings, and be present in the moment. Start by telling them all to quietly focus on the color yellow. Notice all of the yellow things around them. Hopefully they notice yellow things they had never paid attention to before. Ask the participants what they noticed when they only looked at yellow things. You may choose to do another color after this, such as blue. Ask, "When you were looking only at yellow things, did you notice the blue things?" When we are mindful, we can pay closer attention to something. Tell them, "Today we want to pay closer attention to ourselves and how we feel in our bodies. When we do this, it can make it easier to identify how we are feeling and to calm ourselves down when we are sad or upset."

2. Next, provide each participant with a piece of white paper and markers or crayons. Participants will draw a picture of themselves and things that make them feel calm or relaxed. Give participants 10–15 minutes to draw their pictures. When they are done, ask a few participants to share their drawings and what makes them feel calm. Congratulate everyone for doing a great job drawing their pictures and identifying things that help them feel calm.

3. Inform the participants they are now going to do an exercise that will make them feel calm. Let them know they can do this exercise anywhere and anytime they are feeling sad, angry, overwhelmed, or nervous. Have everyone find a comfortable seat. If you decide to play background music, you may start it at this time.

4. Walk the participants through the following guided meditation on the hand-out. You may also choose to give copies of the meditation to participants so they can take it home and do it with their guardian/parents:

5. Invite the participants back into their current surroundings. Ask the following questions:

   ◦ Could you feel the sun shining on you?
   ◦ Could you imagine the wind blowing?
   ◦ Could you hear the leaves crunching in the forest?
   ◦ Did you imagine what it felt like to have raindrops sprinkling on you?
   ◦ Tell me about the rainbow you saw.

○ What things did you imagine surrounding you when I said all of the colors of the rainbow?

Invite a variety of responses from the participants so they have an opportunity to process the meditation. When you have completed the discussion, move on to the opinion questions.

Opinion Questions:

- How would you define mindfulness?

- When can you use this exercise to help you calm down?

Lesson 24 Handout

Meditation

Close your eyes and take a deep breath. Breathe in slowly through your nose, and then exhale your breath out of your mouth. Do this several times. Breathe in, breathe out. In through the nose, and out through the mouth. Now in your mind, picture yourself walking outside. You can feel the warm sun on your skin as your feet hit the pavement. You can feel a light breeze and you hear the tree leaves rustle in the wind. You stop walking for a minute to feel the sunshine on your face and the breeze on your neck. You take a deep breath in through your nose, smelling flowers, and breath out through your mouth.

You continue to walk outside. As you walk you notice a few clouds in the sky and wonder if it might rain. You feel a few cool sprinkles on your skin, which feels nice on this warm day. You continue to walk along the pavement and with each step you breathe in through your nose, and out through your mouth. Breathe in, breathe out. You walk until you see a forest with lots of trees. You decide to walk through the forest as the rain starts to come down and you take cover under the tall trees. Every-thing around you is green. You hear the leaves crunch beneath your feet as you walk. With each crunch you breathe in through your nose, and out through your mouth.

Crunch. Crunch. Crunch.

You walk a short distance through the forest, then come to a clearing and you see a playground. It is still raining, but you decided to walk over to a swing and sit down. On the swing you use your legs and start to pump. Feeling the rain on your face, you take a deep breath in through your nose as the swing goes up, and breathe out through your mouth as you go down. Up and down, breathing in and out. In and out.

As you stop swinging, the rain stops too. You look up and see a rainbow. Each color reminds you of one of your favorite things. Think of some of your favorite things as I say each color. Red… Orange… Yellow… Green… Blue… Purple… Imagine all of your favorite things surrounding you. Take in one last breath, and breathe it out slowly.

When you're ready, open your eyes.

LESSON 25:
Glitter Feelings to Sprinkling Big Emotions

Rationale:

Working through big emotions like anger, jealousy, and sadness can be difficult for children. They may struggle to identify these emotions. Coping and working through big emotions can be even more difficult. Sometimes, the inability to have the coping skills to work through big emotions leads to fits and tantrums for children. This lesson will offer a coping skill for children to help calm their big emotions.

Objectives:

- To identify a coping strategy for big emotions
- To explain a strategy for calming down when upset

Modification for Parents/Guardians:

If this is an effective coping skill for your child, you may choose to carry their calming bottle with you when you are out, to help effectively deal with big emotions. Talk with your child about other ways to deal with big emotions too, and help them identify a variety of coping skills. At home you could make a "calm" basket so your child knows where to find coping skills whenever they are feeling angry, jealous, or sad.

Materials:

- Chart paper

- Marker
- Empty water bottles
- Glitter glue
- Hot water
- Lesson 25 Handout on page 125
- Optional:
  - Food coloring
  - Sequins
  - Super Glue
  - Guided meditation/music

Lesson Plan:

1. Introduce today's lesson by asking everyone to take a big breath and then slowly let it out. Tell the group, "Taking a big breath can help us calm down when we are feeling angry, sad, upset, or even too excited." Then ask the group, "How are you feeling today?" Elicit a few responses from participants.

2. Ask the participants, "Do you ever get sad or angry?" Then follow up with, "What do you do when you are very sad or angry?" Elicit all responses. Tell the participants when we work through our emotions and problems it is called using a coping skill. Ask, "What other coping skills can you think of?" Write their responses on a piece of chart paper labeled "Coping Skills." Make sure to include "taking a deep breath," and refer back to the opening of this lesson and Lesson #24.

3. Tell the participants they are going to make a coping skill today that will help them calm down when they are experiencing big emotions.

4. Give each participant an empty water bottle. Make sure the labels have been removed. Help the participants fill the empty bottle half full with warm water. Squirt glitter glue into the bottle. Be sure to squirt it directly into the water. (If you squirt it on the sides of the bottle the glue may stick and not rub off.) Add optional sequins. Add one drop of optional food coloring. Finish filling the water bottle with hot water. Help the participants tightly secure the bottle cap. Use optional Super Glue (done by a trusted adult) to secure the lid. Shake the bottle up and down so the glitter mixes up in the water.

5. When the project is complete, ask each participant to shake their bottle and then set it down in front of them. Tell participants to take a deep breath in and then slowly and exhale, just like when they started the lesson. Have them continue to inhale and exhale until every last bit of glitter settles. You may also choose to read a guided meditation such as from Lesson 24 Handout on page 119 during this time, or have music playing.

6. Once everyone has had an opportunity to breathe with their glitter bottles, ask if they'd like to do it again. Once you have finished, proceed to the opinion questions to reflect on the lesson.

7. When you have finished the opinion questions, give each participant a hand-out so they can remember additional coping skills when they need them.

Opinion Questions:

- What is a coping skill?
- Did you feel calmer as you took a deep breath in and out?
- How can an adult help you calm down?
- How do you think the glitter bottle will help you calm down?

Lesson 25 Handout

Coping Skills

- Color a picture.

- Sing a song.

- Take a nap.

- Talk to a trusted adult.

- Go for a walk.

- Make a friendship bracelet.

- Drink water and eat a snack.

- Hug your favorite stuffed animal.

- Read a book.

- Dance.

SEX EDUCATION PERMISSION SLIP

Research indicates that sex education promotes comfort and awareness of body, increased self-esteem, and prevention of sexual abuse. As part of our curriculum, we will be discussing sexual health in class. Students will learn about body, identity, communication, diversity, and emotions. Lessons will be implemented from *Colors of You* by Kristen Lilla and Christian Hoeger.

The curriculum was intentionally created for youth and is comprehensive, medically accurate, and age appropriate. In addition, the lesson plans will help your child feel more confident and comfortable in their body, expressing emotions, identifying feelings, and promoting diversity and inclusion.

Students are encouraged to continue the dialogue at home with their parents/guardians. Parent/guardian modifications are included throughout the curriculum and they will be sent home by request.

While we want to provide a well-rounded education for your child, attending the sexual health curriculum is optional. Parents/guardians have the right to have their child participate or opt out of these classes. Please return the permission slip below indicating your decision. If you need additional information, or an outline of the curriculum, please do not hesitate to reach out.

_____

Name of student

I **DO** want my child to participate in *Colors of You*

_____   _____

Signature of parent/guardian   *date*

I **DO NOT** want my child to participate in *Colors of You*

_____   _____

Signature of parent/guardian   *date*

REFERENCES

Ardiel, E. & Rankin, C. (2010). The importance of touch in development. *Paediatr Child Health*, 15(3), 153–156.

Bergman, S.B. (2015). *A Princess Of Great Daring*. Flamingo Rampant.

Bergman, S.B. (2015). *Is That Boy or a Girl?* Flamingo Rampant.

Center for Sex Education. (2020). *Orientation: Teaching about identity, attraction, & behavior*. Morristown, NJ: The Center for Sex Education.

DePaola, T. (1979). *Oliver Button is a Sissy*. Orlando, FL: Harcourt Brace & Company.

Devenny, J. (2021). *Race Cars: A children's book about white privilege*. Beverly, MA: Frances Lincoln Children's Books.

Garcia, G. (2017). *Listening to my Body, 2nd Edition*. Austin, TX: Skinned Knee Publishing.

Goldfarb, E. & Lieberman, L. (2021). Three Decades of Research: The Case for Comprehensive Sex Education. *Journal of Adolescent Health*, 68 (2021), 13–27.

Haffner, D. (2008). *From diapers to Dating: A parent's guide to raising sexually healthy children from infancy to middle school, 2nd Edition*. New York, NY: William Morrow Paperbacks.

Herman, J., Flores, A., & O'Neill, K. (2022). *How Many Adults and Youth Identify as Transgender in the United States?* Los Angeles, CA: The Williams Institute.

Hoeger, C & Lilla, K. (2019). *Vaginas and Periods 101: A Pop-up book*. Omaha, NE: Sex Ed Talk LLC.

Hoffman, S. (2014). *Jacob's New Dress*. Park Ridge, IL: Albert Whitman and Company.

Intersex Society of North American. (2023). *What is Intersex?* Retrieved from https://isna.org/faq/what_is_intersex/

Jennings, J. & Herthel, J. (2014). *I am Jazz*. New York, NY: Dial Books.

Jewell, T. (2020). *This book is Anti-racist: 20 lessons on how to wake up, take action, and do the work.* Beverly, MA: Frances Lincoln Children's Books.

Kamma, A. (2004) *If You Lived when There was Slavery in America.* New York, NY: Scholastic.

Maguire, N. (2020). *My Body Sends a Signal: Helping kids recognize emotions and express feelings.* Hamburg, Germany: Maguire Books.

Martin, C. & Ruble, D. (2010). Patterns of gender and development. *Annual Review of Psychology,* 61, 353–381.

Munsch, R. (1980). *The Paper Bag Princess.* Toronto, CA: Annick Press Ltd.

Office on Women's Health. (2019). *Body Image.* Retrieved from https://www.womenshealth.gov/mental-health/body-image-and-mental-health/body-image#13

Ortner, N. (2018). *My Magic Breath: Finding calm through mindful breathing.* New York, NY: Harper Collins.

Richardson J. & Parnell, P. (2015). *And Tango Makes Three.* New York, NY: Little Simon

Pintor-Carnagey, M. (2023). Sex Positive Families. https://sexpositivefamilies.com

Pintor-Carnagey, M. (2020). Sex Positive Talks to Have with Kids: A guide to raising sexually healthy, informed, empowered young people. Independently published.

Roffman, D. (2012). *Talk to Me First: Everything you need to know to become your kids' "go-to" person about sex.* Boston, MA: Da Capo Lifelong Books.

Roffman, D. (2021). *The Science Of Babies: A little book for big questions about bodies, birth and families.* Vancouver, BC: Birdhouse Kids Media Ltd.

Silverberg, C. (2012). *What Makes a Baby.* New York, NY: Seven Stories Press.

Silverberg, C. (2015). *Sex is a Funny Word: A book about bodies, feelings, and YOU.* New York, NY: Seven Stories Press.

St. John, L. (2019). *Read Me: A parental primer for "the talk."* The MamaSutra Publishing.

Wright, L. (2016). *I Can Handle It.* Calgary, AB: Laurie Wright.

ABOUT THE AUTHORS

Kristen Lilla (she/they) is a Licensed Clinical Social Worker and an AASECT Certified Sex Therapist, Educator, and Supervisor. In 2020, Kristen won the AASECT Sexuality Educator Award. Kristen is also the author of *Boxes and How We Fill Them: A Basic Guide to Sexual Awareness,* and co-author of *Vaginas and Periods 101: A Pop-Up Book.* In addition, Kristen has been quoted in numerous articles from *Cosmopolitan* to CNN. Kristen is an international speaker and has a private practice doing therapy with couples and individuals. When not writing, Kristen loves to travel, shop, and sip on a hot latte.

Christian Hoeger (she/her) is a Licensed Mental Health Practitioner in the state of Nebraska, after earning her Masters of Arts and Masters of Education in Psychological Counseling from Teachers College, Columbia University. She is the former Director of Counseling at Girls Inc. of Omaha but is now focusing full-time on her private practice in which she specializes in working with the LGBTQ+ community, teens, and complex post-traumatic stress disorder (CPTSD). Christian has presented at the National Sex Education Conference several times, has published lessons by the Center for Sex Education, and is the co-author of *Vaginas and Periods 101: A Pop-Up Book.* In her free time, she is raising feminist twin boys, being a local foodie, and looking for her next scuba diving adventure.

• • •

SEX ED
TALK

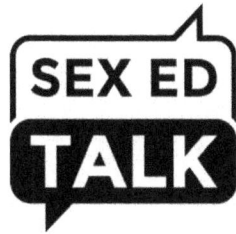

www.SexEdTalk.com